Ultrasound Imaging - Current Topics

Edited by Felix Okechukwu Erondu

Published in London, United Kingdom

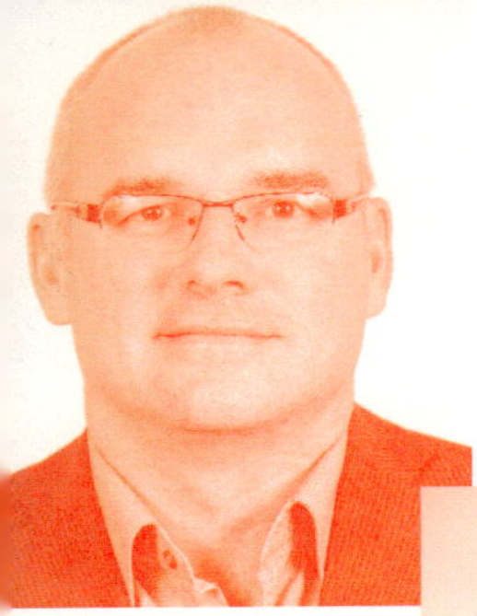
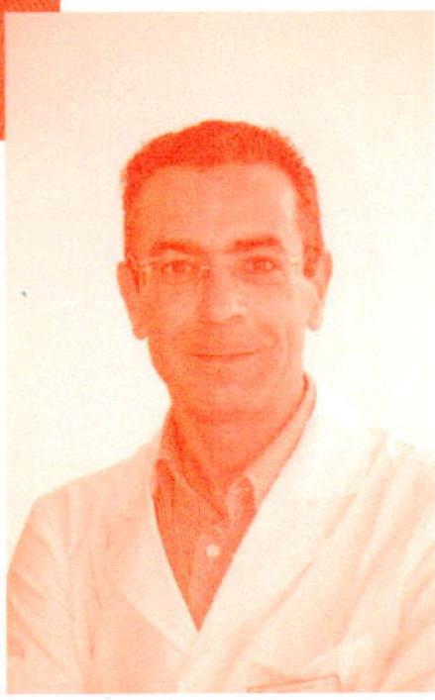
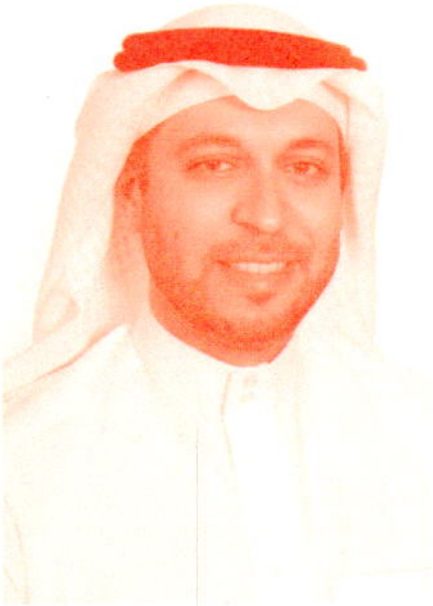
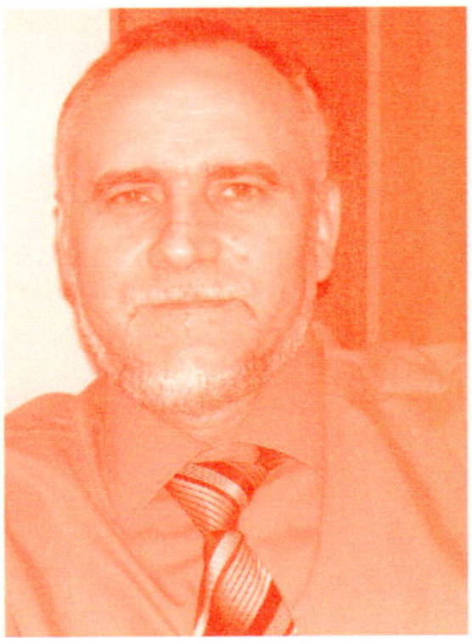
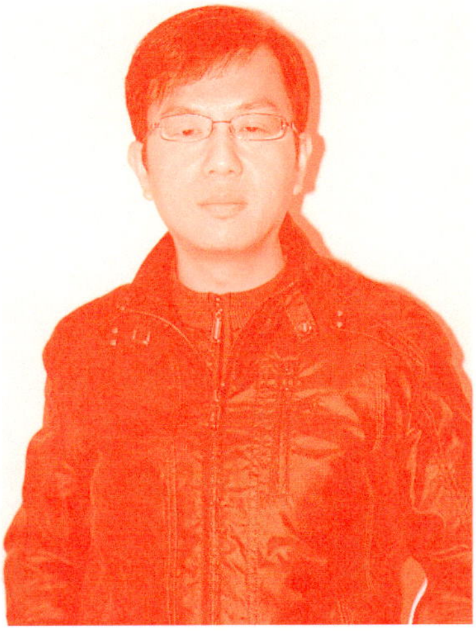
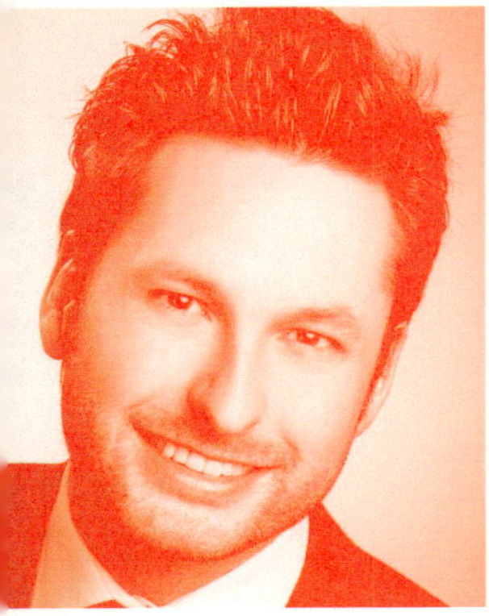
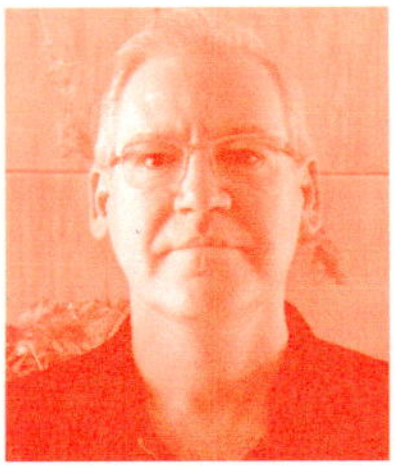

IntechOpen

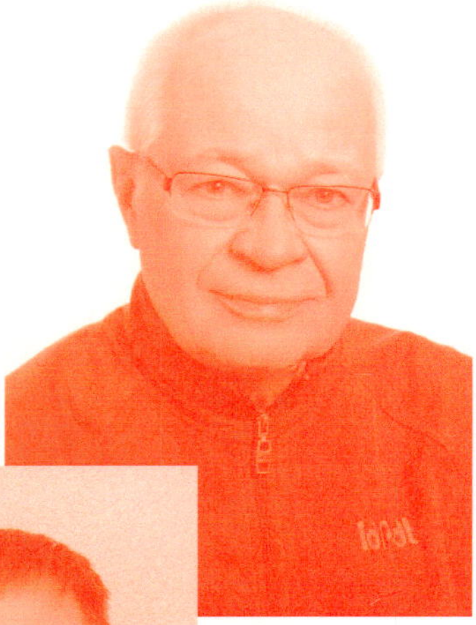
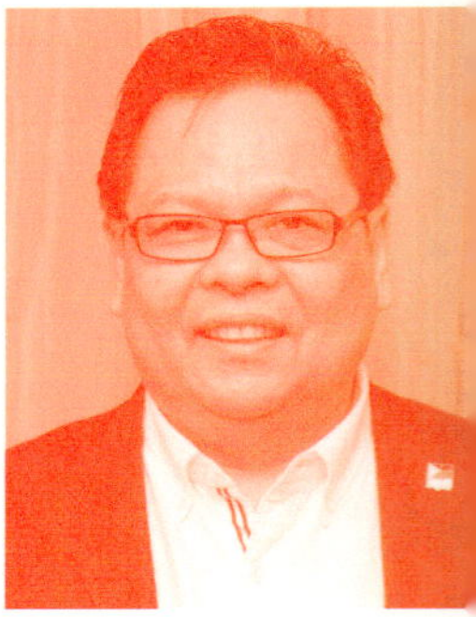
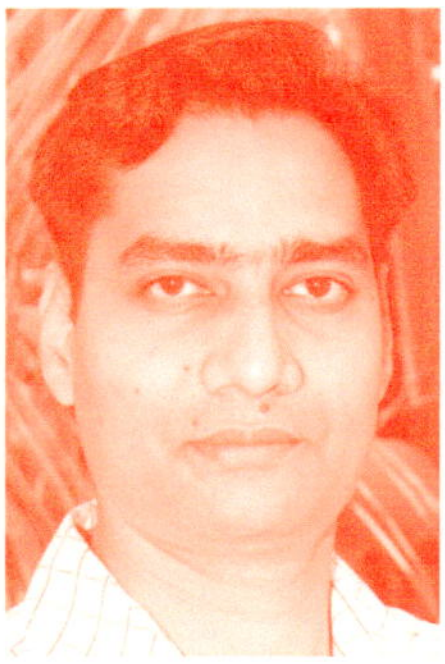
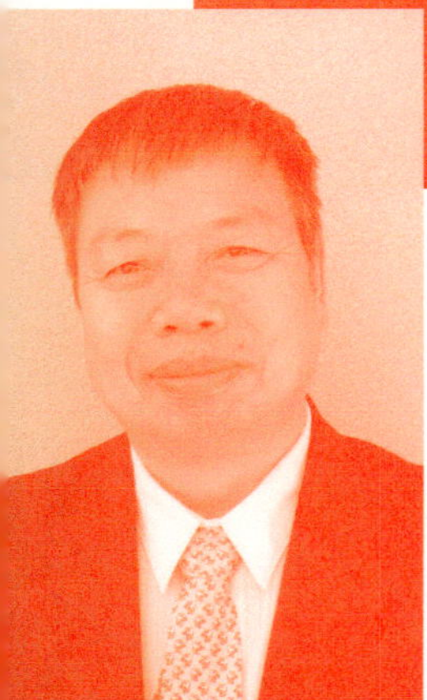
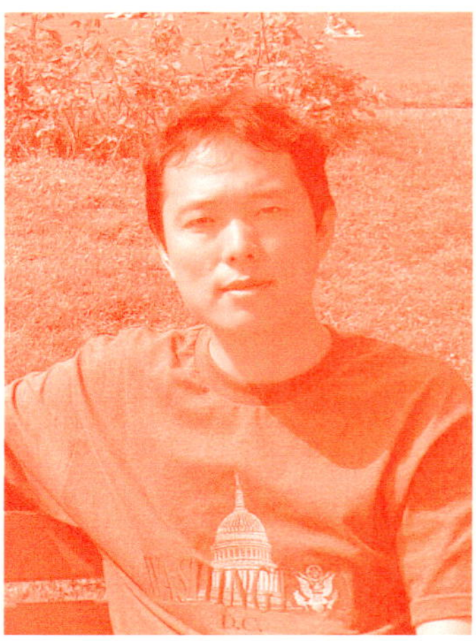
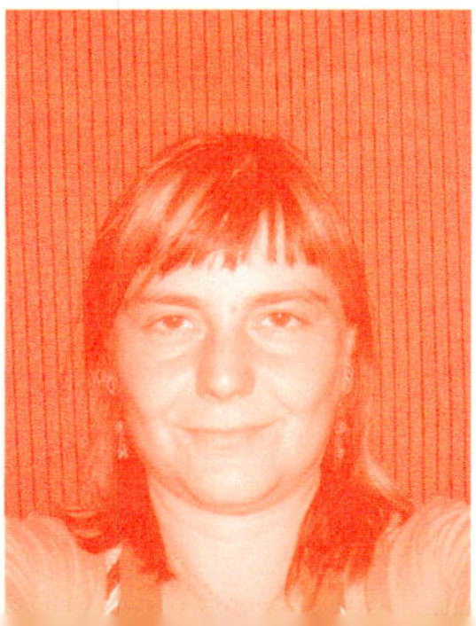

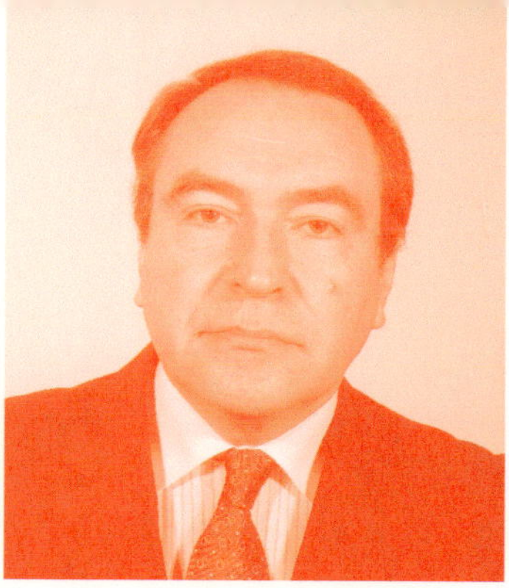

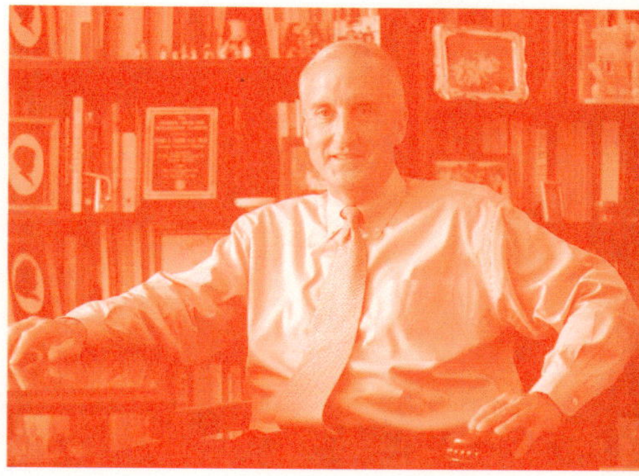

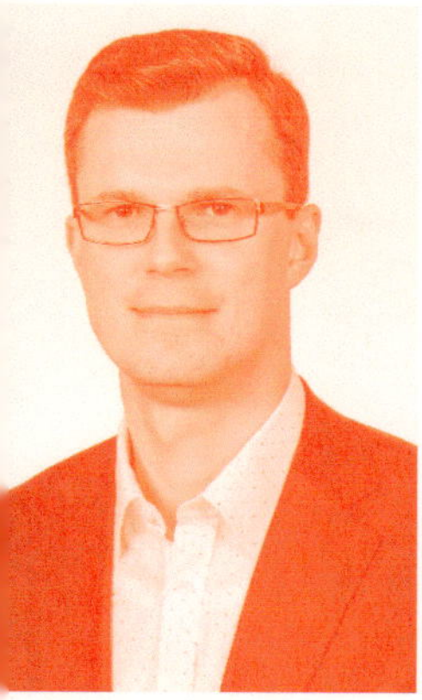

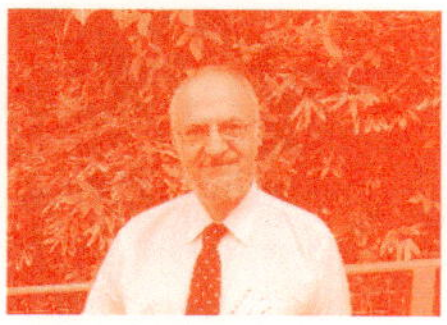

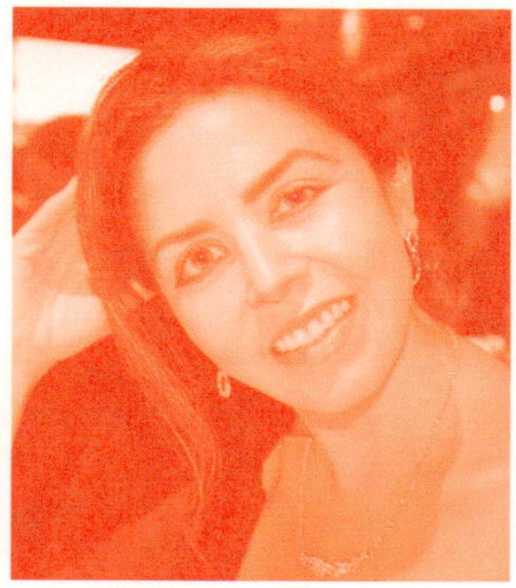

Supporting open minds since 2005

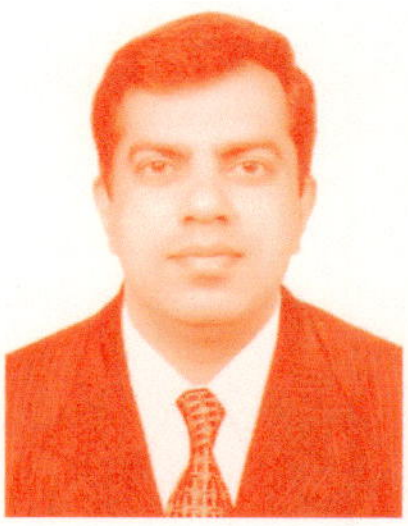

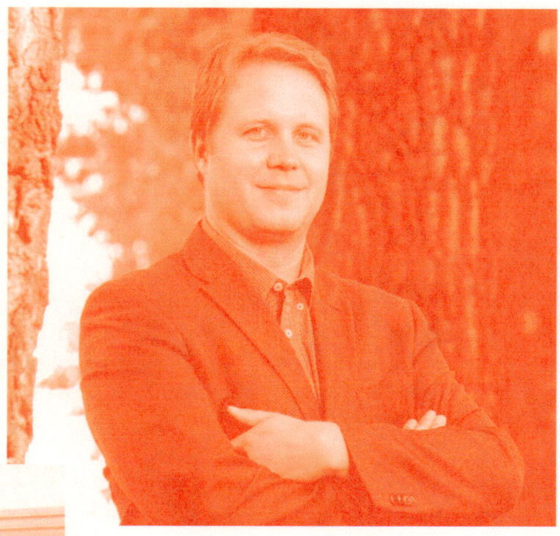

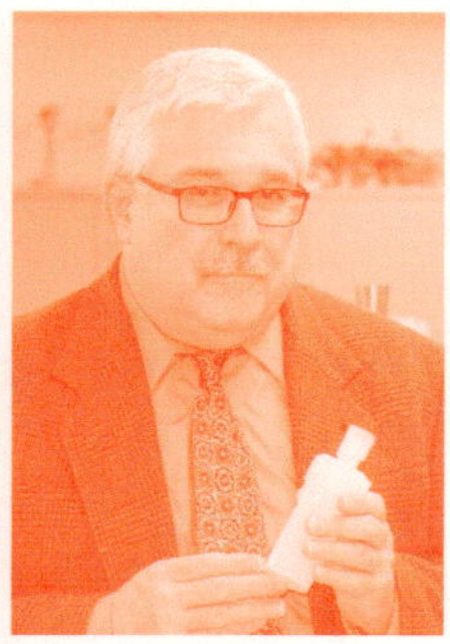

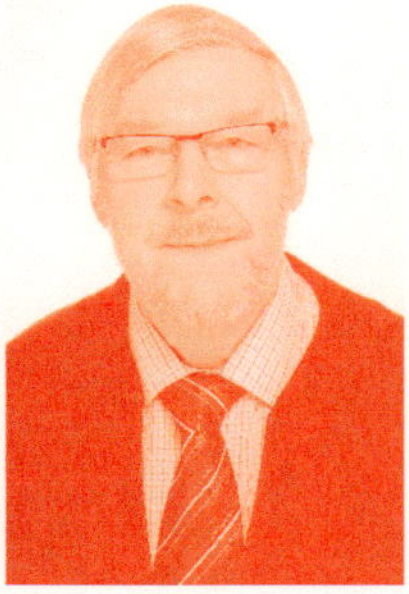

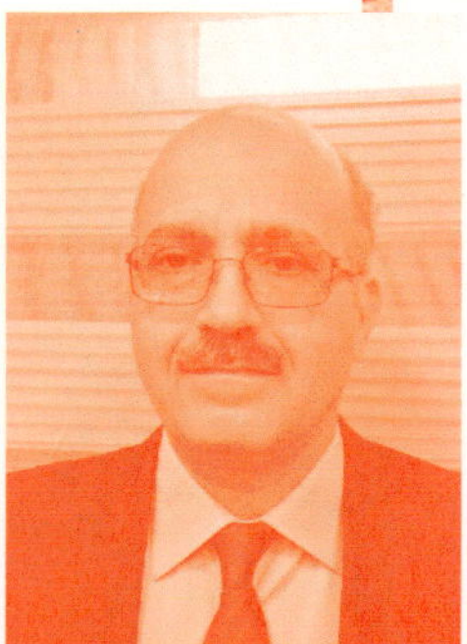

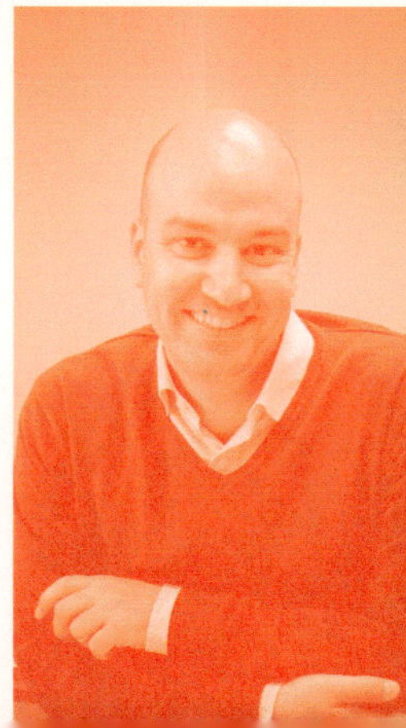

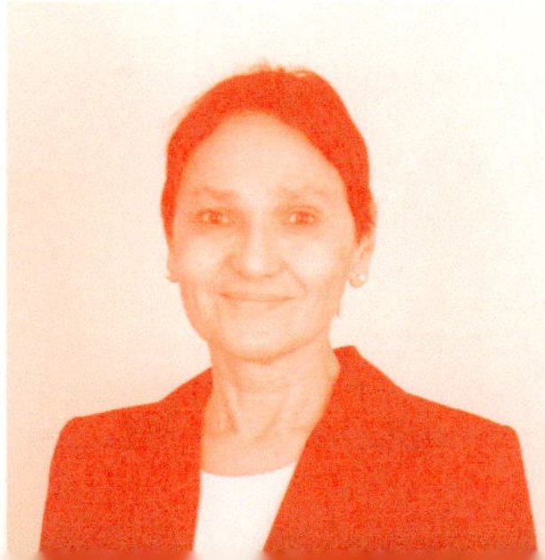

Ultrasound Imaging - Current Topics
http://dx.doi.org/10.5772/intechopen.95178
Edited by Felix Okechukwu Erondu

Contributors
Florentin Ananu Vreju, Ștefan Cristian Dinescu, Răzvan Adrian Ionescu, Horațiu Valeriu Popoviciu, Claudiu Avram, Solomon Demissie, Yonas Derso, Mulatie Atalay, Jong Hwa Lee, Jae Uk Lee, Seung Wan Yoo, Arthur Fleischer, Sai Chennupati, Ercan Ayaz, María Eugenia Aponte-Rueda, María Isabel de Abreu, Haithem Zaafouri, Meryam Mesbahi, Nizar Khedhiri, Wassim Riahi, Mouna Cherif, Dhafer Haddad, Anis Ben Maamer, J.M. López-Alvarez, O. Pérez Quevedo, S. Alonso-Graña López-Manteola, J.F. Loro Ferrer, J. Naya- Esteban, D.L. Lorenzo-Villegas, Felix Okechukwu Erondu

First published in London, United Kingdom, 2022 by IntechOpen
IntechOpen is the global imprint of INTECHOPEN LIMITED, registered in England and Wales, registration number: 11086078, 5 Princes Gate Court, London, SW7 2QJ, United Kingdom
Printed in Croatia

British Library Cataloguing-in-Publication Data
A catalogue record for this book is available from the British Library

Additional hard and PDF copies can be obtained from orders@intechopen.com

Ultrasound Imaging - Current Topics
Edited by Felix Okechukwu Erondu
p. cm.
Print ISBN 978-1-78984-877-9
Online ISBN 978-1-78985-186-1
eBook (PDF) ISBN 978-1-78985-331-5

For EU product safety concerns:
IN TECH d.o.o., Prolaz Marije Krucifikse Kozulić 3, 51000 Rijeka, Croatia, info@intechopen.com or visit our website at intechopen.com.

Meet the editor

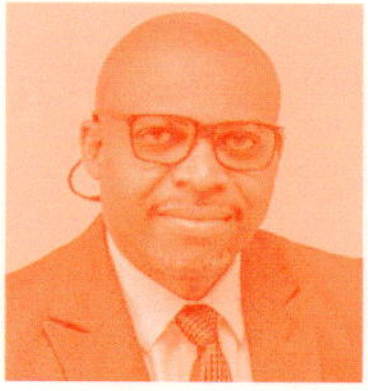

Felix Okechukwu Erondu is a Professor of Radiography and Dean of the Faculty of Health Sciences, College of Medicine and Health Sciences, Gregory University Uturu, Nigeria. He is also a practicing medical imaging consultant with more than 25 years of clinical experience. He is an expert in ultrasound and medical imaging and a mentor for both undergraduate and post-graduate students. He has authored five textbooks and more than sixty scientific publications in rated, peer-reviewed journals. He is the founder and CEO of Image Diagnostics Inc., a chain of diagnostic facilities located in various states of Nigeria.

Contents

Preface

Ultrasound technology has revolutionized the way medicine is practiced by providing an easy-to-use, available, cost-effective, and non-invasive means of making diagnoses. It complements other methods of physical examination such as palpation, visual inspection, auscultation, and percussion. This book, *Ultrasound Imaging - Current Topics* is a hybrid resource capturing current topics in ultrasound imaging and CT scanning. It highlights contemporary topics in what would otherwise be considered a well-researched discipline.

The book begins with a review of anatomy and dimensional variations in major organs like the spleen, and further highlights the use of ultrasound in pediatric gastrointestinal emergencies. It goes on to describe the applications of ultrasound in the evaluation of musculoskeletal disorders and nerve imaging, training models, and the newer concepts of molecular sonography.

The book explains complex topics from the viewpoint of experienced authors, thus making it indispensable for individuals desiring both clinical and theoretical information. It is written in simple, easy-to-understand language and has appeal to those looking for additional resources in the diverse field of ultrasound imaging.

As a compendium of scientific evolution in ultrasound imaging, this book is recommended for students and practitioners alike.

Felix Okechukwu Erondu
Department of Radiography and Radiation Sciences,
Gregory University,
Uturu, Abia State, Nigeria

Chapter 1

Anatomy, Sonographic Features, and Dimensional Variations of Spleen among Individuals with Different Sociodemographic and Anthropometric Measurement

Solomon Demissie, Mulatie Atalay and Yonas Derso

Abstract

The spleen is a vital lymphoid soft organ located in the left hypochondrium region. It is a multi-dimensional organ that enlarges in all dimensions during some disease conditions. Recently, splenomegaly prevalence has been increasing throughout the world. Due to the lack of attention in clinical practice, splenomegaly has become quite a common problem in all parts of the world. The detection of the spleen by palpation is not approval of enlarged spleen because normal spleen may be palpable. A detailed knowledge of morphometric variations of the spleen is of great value in diagnosing splenomegaly clinically, radiologically, and for surgical procedures. Measurement of spleen size by sonography is important as it gives true result than splenic palpation and for identification of disorders present with enlargement or reduction of the spleen. Therefore, this study aimed to assess the anatomy, sonography, and dimensional variation of spleen among individuals with different sociodemographic and anthropometric measurements. The current study reviews different types of literature conducted on spleen all over the world. The result from overall spleen dimensions review shows measurements vary: spleen length (7–14 cm), spleen width (2–7.5 cm), spleen thickness (2–7 cm), and spleen volume (20–350 cm^3). The literature revealed that spleen dimensions are affected by geographical differences, races, nutritional status, physical exercise, and anthropometric measurements. The result from reviews shows that spleen dimensions are larger in males than females. As age increases, spleen dimensions significantly decrease. Spleen dimensions positively correlate with height, weight, body mass index, and body surface of individuals. The spleen dimensions were higher in males than in females and have significant positive correlation with height, weight, body mass index, and body surface area. Clinicians, radiologists, and surgeons should confirm splenomegaly by both palpation and sonography. Spleen dimensions variation due to geographical sex, age, and other anthropometric measurements should be taken into consideration during their clinical investigation. Radiologists should measure all dimensions of spleen rather than the length to rule out splenomegaly correctly.

Keywords: spleen, anatomy, sonography, dimensional variation

1. Introduction

The spleen is the largest lymphoid soft organ that lies in the left hypochondrium between the fundus of the stomach and the diaphragm [1]. Its long axis extends from 9th to 11th ribs on the left side with its long axis running parallel to the 10th rib (**Figure 1**) [2].

The shape of the spleen is ovoid-like pulpy mass about the size + shape of one's fist with a convex outer diaphragmatic surface and an indented inner visceral surface [3]. The diaphragmatic surface of spleen is convex and smooth to fit the concavity of the diaphragm, while the visceral surface is irregular and related to the stomach, left kidney, left suprarenal gland, and left colic flexure [4]. The medial end (apex) lies in line with the spine of 10th thoracic vertebra about 4 cm from the midline, and the lateral end (base) does not descend beyond the midaxillary line [5].

The functions of the spleen are centered on the systemic circulation [6]. It contains two functionally and morphologically distinct compartments: the red pulp and the white pulp. The red pulp functions as a blood filter that removes foreign material and damaged erythrocytes, and the white pulp initiates immune responses to blood-borne antigens (**Figure 2**) [7].

The spleen is involved and enlarged in a variety of clinical conditions. Its size is mostly affected by infections, hematological disorders, infiltrative states, and immunological and malignant diseases [8, 9]. A variety of diseases condition alters spleen dimensions, where splenomegaly and its consequence become a primary clinical concern in developing countries [10]. It is commonly seen in about 63% of patients with pulmonary arterial hypertension [11], infectious mononucleosis [12], malaria [13], lymphoma [14], kala-azar [15], typhoid fever [16], liver disease (hepatitis and cirrhosis) [17], hematological diseases, metabolism diseases, and cancer [18]. The altered splenic dimensions and structure during these diseases result in asymptomatic enlargement and complications such as hematoma formation, rupture, hypersplenism, ectopic spleen, and torsion that affect other adjacent organs [19].

Splenic atrophy is also another common problem seen in diseases like sickle cell anemia, where progressive atrophy as a result of repeated attacks of vaso-occlusion and infarction caused by these diseases leads to auto splenectomy [20].

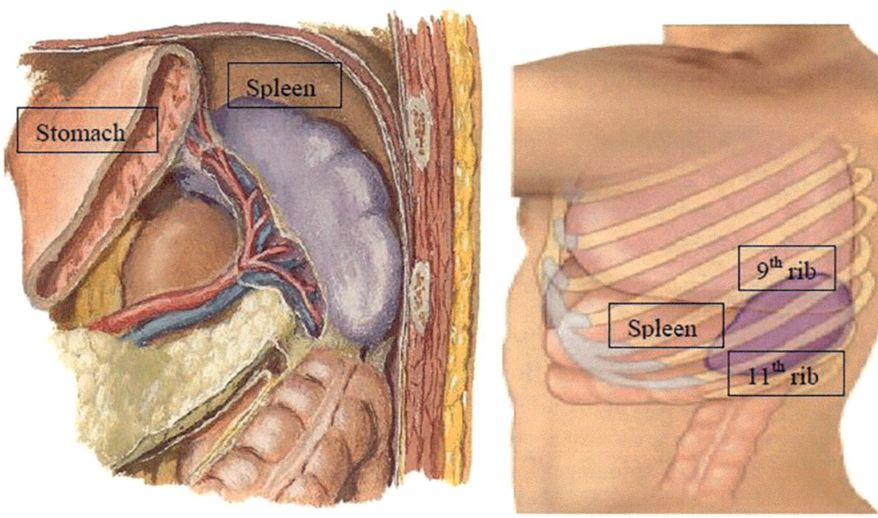

Figure 1.
Spleen anatomical location.

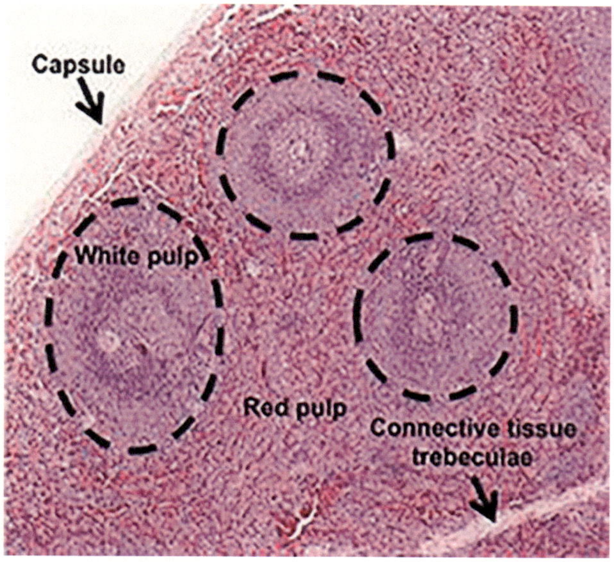

Figure 2.
Spleen histological features.

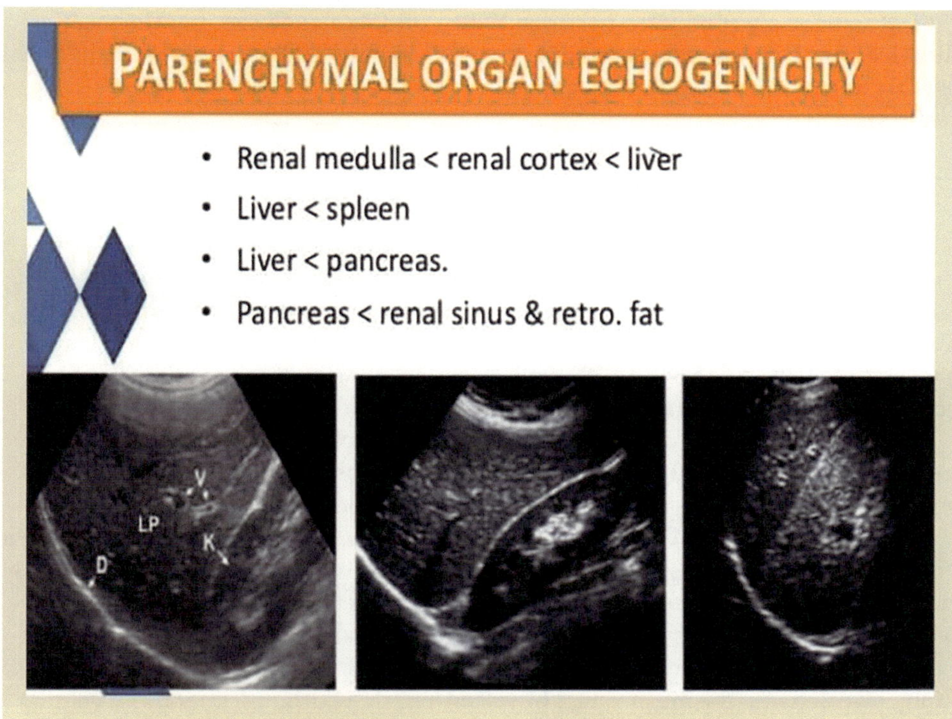

Figure 3.
Spleen sonographic comparison with kidney and liver.

The dimension of the spleen is evaluated using conventional radiography, ultrasonography, scintigraphy, computed tomography, and magnetic resonance imaging [21]. However, ultrasonography is a non-invasive, safe, quick, and accurate method for measurement of spleen size [22]. On sonography spleen is characterized as crescent-shaped with outer convexity is smooth, whereas the inner margin is indented. Its echo structure is homogeneous and more echogenic than healthy liver tissue and markedly hyperechoic compared to kidney tissue (**Figure 3**) [23].

The average dimensions of the spleen are 12.5 cm, 7.5 cm, and 2.5 cm in length, width, and thickness, respectively, and 150–200 g in weight, but its dimensions vary considerably [20]. The literature revealed that spleen dimensions are affected by geographical differences, races, nutritional status, and anthropometric measurements [21–23]. The following are types of literature reviewed.

2. Literature reviews

2.1 Overall morph metric evaluation of normal dimension of spleen

Average overall dimension of spleen varies from race to race and region to region. The study designed to evaluate splenic size by ultrasonography (US) of healthy Turkish men found the average splenic length to be 10.76 (±1.84) cm [24]. Study conducted in Istanbul Turkey found that the mean spleen volume (SV), splenic length (SL), width (SW), and thickness (ST) were 198 (±88) cm^3, 9.96 (±2.1) cm, 8.87 (±1.6) cm, and 4.58 (±0.8) cm, respectively [25]. In another study conducted on North Indian adult population, splenic dimensions were 10.67 (±1.62) cm in length, 6.26 (±1.66) cm in width, and 4.86 (±1.22) cm in thickness [26]. Recent study conducted in North West Ethiopia also found that the mean dimensions of spleen, the mean splenic length, width, thickness, and volume with (±SD), were 9.95 cm (±1.12), 4.3 cm (±0.7), 3.8 cm (±0.8), and 92.0(±38.4) cm^3, respectively [27].

2.2 Normal spleen dimensions in correlation with sex

Different literature states that spleen dimension varies in relation to sex, with more studies indicating that males have larger spleen dimensions than females. Ultrasound assessment of spleen size in collegiate athletes conducted in Kentucky, USA, shows that spleen length and width (cm) 9.91 (±1.27) cm, 4.74 (±0.91) cm and 11.29 (±1.49) cm, 5.54 (±1.28) cm in female and male, respectively. The study concludes that men have larger spleen size than females [28].

In a study conducted on Saudi Arabian adult, the average splenic volume of males was 196.95 (±48.70) cm^3 and that of females was 196.95 (±26.97) cm^3. The study concludes that a significant difference was found between sex [29].

In a study conducted on sonological evaluation of the spleen in an adult Southern Nigerian population, lengths of the spleen were 9.62 (±1) cm and 9.12 (±1.22) cm for the males and females, respectively. A significant difference ($p < 0.05$) was found between the sex, and it is significantly larger in the males [30].

Measurement of normal spleen dimensions in adult Sudanese using ultrasonography revealed that the mean values of spleen length, width, thickness, and volume were 10.3 (±1.2), 3.3 (±0.4), 3.9 (±0.6), and 73.3 (±23) respectively for males and 9.2 (±0.9), 3.1 (±0.3), 3.6 (±0.6), and 56.5 (±18.0) respectively for female. The study concludes that men have larger spleens than females in relation of spleens to sex [31].

2.3 Normal spleen dimensions in correlation with age

The study conducted in Pakistan to determine the normal spleen parameters in adults shows that the mean spleen sizes of the participants were 9.81 ± 1.73 cm, and a significant positive correlation was observed between age and spleen size of the individuals ($r = 0.053$, $p = 0.012$) [32].

The splenic dimension study conducted in Western Nepal revealed that in age groups of 16–30, 31–45, 46–60, and 61–75 years, respectively, revealed that spleen length for males (10.07 ± 0.7 cm, 10.1 ± 0.54 cm, 9.5 ± 0.7 cm, and 9.0 ± 0.43 cm, respectively) and for the females (9.83 ± 0.53 cm, 9.58 ± 0.58 cm, 9.2 ± 0.64 cm, and 8.8 ± 0.36 cm, respectively). The spleen thickness for males (4.1 ± 0.5 cm, 4.05 ± 0.58 cm, 3.43 ± 0.38 cm, and 3.0 ± 0.36 cm, respectively) and for the females (4.06 ± 0.47 cm, 3.78 ± 0.48 cm, 3.38 ± 0.35 cm, and 2.29 ± 0.23 cm, respectively). The results show that the splenic length and thickness decreased with increase in age in both males and females [33].

In a study conducted on adults of Tripura, India, with age groups of (15–30 years), (31–45 years), (46–60 years), (61–75 years), and (>75 years), the spleen lengths were 9.00 ± 1.07 cm, 8.79 ± 1.44, 9.15 ± 1.04, 8.63 ± 1.55, and 7.64 ± 1.06 cm, respectively. Correlation analysis showed that spleen length was negatively correlated with age in all adults. So, with increasing age, spleen length was found to be decreasing, which is significant ($p < 0.05$) [34].

A study conducted to establish the normal range of the splenic dimensions in North Indian adult population revealed that the splenic length, width, and thickness decreased with increase in age in both males and females. The results show that in both males and females, the splenic length decreased at a slow rate up to the age of 50 years, after which it decreased rapidly; the splenic width decreased with age up to 30 years; thereafter, it remained relatively constant up to the age of 50 years and after that the splenic width decreased. It also shows that in both males and females, splenic thickness was constant up to the age of 50 years, after which there was a fall in the splenic thickness [35].

The studies from Rajasthan, India, revealed that the length was 8.69 ± 0.93 cm in adults and 9.64 ± 0.64 cm in older subjects. The width was 3.59 ± 0.55 cm in adults, while in older subjects, the width was 3.38 ± 0.38 cm [36].

2.4 Normal spleen dimensions in correlation with height, weight, BSA, and BMI

In a study conducted in Saudi in Jordanian population, ultra-sonographic assessment of splenic volume revealed that splenic dimensions were 10.72 ± 1.37 cm in length, 7.40 ± 1.52 cm in width, 4.40 ± 1.47 cm in depth, and 184.15 ± 79.56 cm^3 in volume. Moderate positive linear relationships were found between the splenic dimension and body height, weight, BSA, and BMI ($r > 0.3$). This correlation was statistically significant ($p < 0.0001$) [37].

Study conducted in the United States revealed that spleen length and volume were associated with body height in which body height alone accounted for 17.3% of spleen length variability and 14.9% of spleen volume variability [38].

Sonographic evaluation of spleen size in athletes conducted in Canada revealed that the mean splenic dimensions were 11.4 ± 1.7 cm length (range, 8.2–16.1 cm), 10.8 ± 1.4 cm width (range, 8–14 cm), 5.0 ± 0.8 cm in thickness, and 333.6 ± 116.1 cm^2 in volume. All splenic measurements correlated better with height than weight [39].

Assessment of dimensions of spleen in normal adult Kashmiri population revealed that the mean length of the spleen was 10.20 + 1.40 cm and the width was 8.63 + 1.57 cm. The study found a statistically significant correlation of splenic dimensions with body weight and BMI [40].

3. Dimensional measurement on sonography

The dimension of spleen is measured as follows.

Spleen length: the maximum distance measured in longitudinal plane at hilum between the dome of the spleen and the splenic tip.

Apparently healthy individual: individuals with no signs and symptoms of disease.

Spleen width: the maximum dimension measured in a plane perpendicular to the length at hilum between the medial and lateral borders of the spleen.

Spleen thickness: the maximum AP dimension measured on the transverse section.

Spleen volume: calculated using the standard ellipsoid formula (length × width × depth × 0.523); this formula is frequently used for estimating the volume of many irregularly shaped organs (**Figures 4–6**) [41].

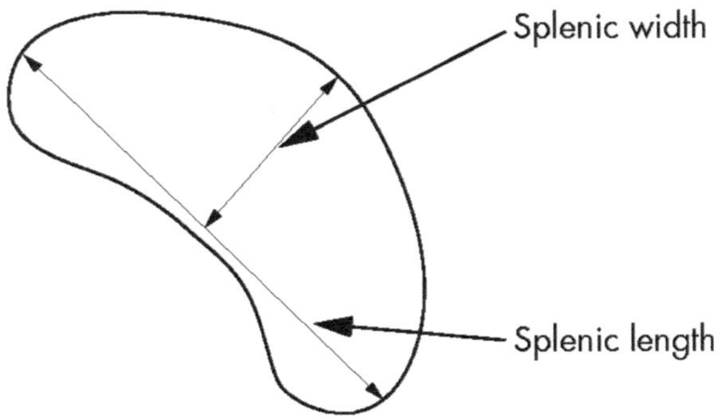

Figure 4.
Spleen length and width measurement.

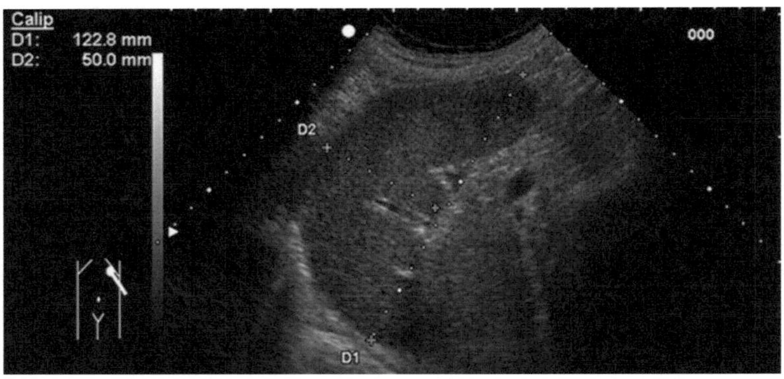

Figure 5.
Spleen sonographic length and width measurement.

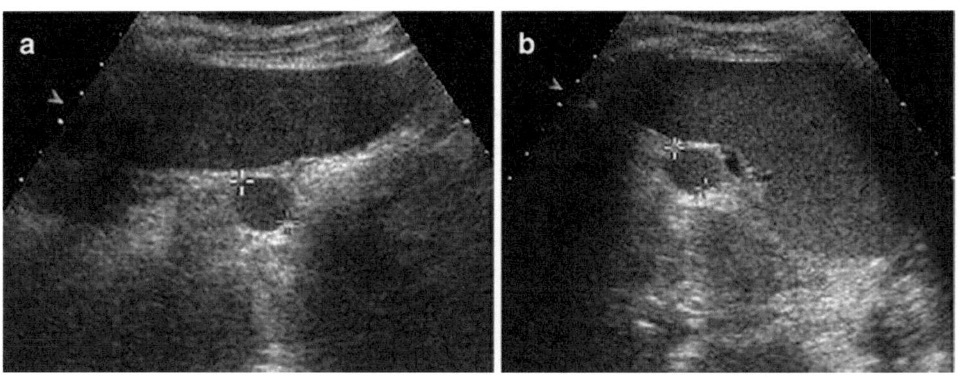

Figure 6.
Spleen thickness sonographic measurement.

4. Discussion

This study describes the morphometry of spleen dimensions and compares the presence of a significant difference between sex and age as well as dimensional correlations with anthropometric measurements. The sonography assessment of spleen dimensions provides essential inputs for clinicians in daily clinical practice for the proper diagnosis of splenomegaly [33, 35, 42]. This study provides estimates of spleen to help radiologists for the diagnosis of diseases related to splenomegaly and atrophy, also used by hematologists and immunologists for the diagnosis of various gastrointestinal and hematological diseases, in addition to forensic studies [43–45].

The result from overall spleen dimensions review shows that measurements vary as follows: spleen length (7–14 cm), spleen width (2–7.5 cm), spleen thickness (2–7 cm), and spleen volume (20–350 cm^3). The average dimensional difference between studies is probably due to age group differences, geographical differences, nutritional status, physical exercise, and race differences, which were stated in different literature [25, 42, 45–48].

In most of studies reviewed, the spleen dimensions were lower in females than males. This is due to histological and genetic differences of spleens between males and females. On histological studies, females have fewer total red cell mass, when compared to males [38, 49]. Studies conducted in Turkey, Saudi, Nigeria, Sudan, and Ethiopia support this idea [30, 31, 45, 50, 51]. But, one study conducted in Egypt showed the length was higher among females than males. This may be due to nutritional status where Egyptian culture recommends women to gain weight for fertility purposes [52, 53].

In most of the study reviewed, as age increases the spleen length, width, thickness, and volume are reduced. This is from the fact that as age increases, the number and size of B cell follicles of the white pulp of the spleen decrease. This implies a decrease of germinal center of spleen, which reduces overall spleen dimension [54–56]. This review is supported by the studies conducted in Iraq, Nepal, and India [33, 35, 36, 42, 57]. But, this summary of review does not agree with the studies conducted in Pakistan, Jordan, and Nigeria [32, 37, 51, 58]. The difference is maybe due to nutritional status where larger anthropometric measurements and obesity were observed in the studies of Pakistan, Jordan, and Nigeria.

Physiological studies indicate that as individual's height, weight, BMI, and BSA increase, the blood volume increases. This increase of blood volume requires larger spleens for filtration. This fact is supported by most of literature reviewed where all dimensions were positively correlated with height, weight, BMI, and BSA. The studies conducted in Jordan, the United States, India, Sudan, and Ethiopia were some of the studies that support this idea [26, 37, 38, 59].

5. Conclusion

This chapter gives baseline information for clinicians as well as for academicians about the morphometric variation of spleen dimensions. Hence, it helps in diagnosing pathological cases associated with spleen, both splenomegaly as well as splenic atrophy. Therefore, clinicians should consider this variation during their diagnosis. Radiology professionals also should measure all dimensions rather than the length alone to rule out splenomegaly correctly.

Funding

No specific funding was received for the study from any organization.

Competing interests

No competing interest.

Consent for publication

Not applicable.

Availability of data and materials

All relevant data are included in the article.

Author details

Solomon Demissie[1*], Mulatie Atalay[1] and Yonas Derso[2]

1 Department of Clinical Anatomy, College of Medicine and Health Science, Arba Minch University, Arba Minch, Ethiopia

2 Department of Physiology, College of Medicine and Health Science, Arba Minch University, Arba Minch, Ethiopia

*Address all correspondence to: soll12162129@gmail.com

References

[1] Singh V. Textbook of Anatomy Abdomen and Lower Limb. Volume II. 2nd ed. India: Elsevier Health Sciences; 2014. 93p.

[2] Sinnatamby CS. Last's Anatomy e-Book: Regional and Applied. 12th ed. India: Elsevier Health Sciences; 2011. 560p.

[3] Nayak BN, Buttar HS. Health benefits of tryptophan in children and adults. Journal of Pharmaceutical Sciences and Technology Management. 2015;**1**:8-12

[4] Chaudhry SR, Panuganti K. Anatomy, Abdomen and Pelivs. Spleen StatPearls Treasure Island (FL): StatPearls Publishing StatPearls Publishing LLC; 2019

[5] Moore K, Dalley I. AF & Agur, AMR Clinically Oriented Anatomy. Philadelphia, Wolters Kluwer Health/ Lippincott Williams & Wilkins; 2014

[6] Haley PJ. The lymphoid system: A review of species differences. Journal of Toxicologic Pathology. 2017;**30**(2): 111-123

[7] Nolte MA, Hamann A, Kraal G, Mebius RE. The strict regulation of lymphocyte migration to splenic white pulp does not involve common homing receptors. Immunology. 2002;**106**(3): 299-307

[8] Levy AD, Mortele KJ, Yeh BM. Gastrointestinal Imaging: Oxford University Press, USA; 2015

[9] Niederau C, Sonnenberg A, Müller J, Erckenbrecht J, Scholten T, Fritsch W. Sonographic measurements of the normal liver, spleen, pancreas, and portal vein. Radiology 1983;**149**(2):537-540

[10] Lv Y, Lau WY, Li Y, Deng J, Han X, Gong X, et al. Hypersplenism: History and current status. Experimental and Therapeutic Medicine. 2016; **12**(4):2377-2382

[11] Tonelli AR, Yadav R, Gupta A, Arrossi AV, Heresi GA, Dweik RA. Spleen size in idiopathic and heritable pulmonary arterial hypertension. Respiration. 2013;**85**(5):391-399

[12] Kinderknecht JJ. Infectious mononucleosis and the spleen. Current Sports Medicine Reports. 2002; **1**(2):116-120

[13] Alkadarou T, Musa A, Alkadarou A, Mahfouz MS, Troye-Blomberg M, Elhassan AM, et al. Immunological characteristics of hyperreactive malarial splenomegaly syndrome in Sudanese patients. Journal of Tropical Medicine. **2013**;2013:1-5

[14] Smeltzer J, Habermann TM, Timucin T, Nagorney D, Ristow K, Colgan JP, et al. Long term clinical outcomes in patients with massive splenomegaly and non-Hodgkin's lymphoma treated with splenectomy American Society of Hematology; 2012;**120**(21):2692

[15] Varma N, Naseem S. Hematologic changes in visceral leishmaniasis/kala azar. Indian Journal of Hematology and Blood Transfusion. 2010;**26**(3):78-82

[16] Sahu N, Rath S, Padhy RN. Role of abdominal ultrasound in the diagnosis of typhoid fever in pediatric patients. Journal of Medical Ultrasound. 2016; **24**(4):150-153

[17] Chapman J, Bansal P, Goyal A, Azevedo AM. Splenomegaly. In: StatPearls. Treasure Island (FL): StatPearls Publishing; 2021. PMID: 28613657

[18] Kienle DL. The spleen in hematologic malignancies.

Therapeutische Umschau Revue Therapeutique. 2013;**70**(3):163-169

[19] Aubrey-Bassler FK, Sowers N. 613 cases of splenic rupture without risk factors or previously diagnosed disease: A systematic review. BMC Emergency Medicine. 2012;**12**(1):1-14

[20] Babadoko A, Ibinaye P, Hassan A, Yusuf R, Ijei I, Aiyekomogbon J, et al. Autosplenectomy of sickle cell disease in Zaria, Nigeria: An ultrasonographic assessment. Oman Medical Journal. 2012;**27**(2):121

[21] Poulin E, Thibault C. The anatomical basis for laparoscopic splenectomy. Canadian Journal of Surgery Journal Canadien de Chirurgie. 1993;**36**(5):484-488

[22] Megremis SD, Vlachonikolis IG, Tsilimigaki AM. Spleen length in childhood with US: Normal values based on age, sex, and somatometric parameters. Radiology 2004;**231**(1): 129-134

[23] Ahmed OF. Ahmed of assesment of normal hepatosplenic span using ultrasound in egyptian population. Natural Sciences. 2017;**15**(8):215-219

[24] Serter S, Ceylan C, Tunçyürek Ö, Örgüç Ş, Pabuçcu Y. Sonographic evaluation of spleen size and prevalence of accessory spleen in a healthy male Turkish population. Turkish Journal of Hematology. 2010;**27**(1):25-28

[25] Caglar V, Alkoc O, Uygur R, Serdaroglu O, Ozen O. Determination of normal splenic volume in relation to age, gender and body habitus: A stereological study on computed tomography. Folia Morphologica. 2014;**73**(3):331-338

[26] Asghar A, Naaz S, Agrawal D, Sharma P. Morphometric study of spleen in North Indian adult population: CT Scan image based study. Journal of Clinical and Diagnostic Research. 2011;**5**(5):974-977

[27] Tekle Y, Gudadhe DR, Abreha M, Muche A, Tegegne Z, Hiware SD. Morphometric assessment of the normal dimensions of the adult spleen in North-west Ethiopia region—A radiological study. Annals of International Medical and Dental Research. 2018;**4**(4):34-37

[28] Hosey RG, Mattacola CG, Kriss V, Armsey T, Quarles J, Jagger J. Ultrasound assessment of spleen size in collegiate athletes. British Journal of Sports Medicine. 2006;**40**(3):251-254

[29] Siddiqui MA, Ali AHA, Bedewi MA, Serhan OO. Estimation of standard splenic volume in Saudi Arabian adult population: Using 3D reconstruction of Abdominal CT scan Images. Open Journal of Internal Medicine. 2014;**4**(01):7

[30] Udoaka A, Enyi C, Agi C. Sonological evaluation of the liver, spleen and the kidneys in an adult southern Nigerian population. Asian Journal of Medical Sciences. 2013; **5**(2):33-36

[31] Yousif JM. Measurement of Normal Spleen in Sudanese by Using Ultrasonography. Sudan: Sudan University of Science and Technology; 2016. 61p

[32] Khan SA, Yasmeen S, Adil H, Adil SO, Huda F, Khan S. Sonographic evaluation of normal liver, spleen, and renal parameters in adult population: A multicenter study. Journal of the College of Physicians and Surgeons Pakistan. 2018;**28**(11):834

[33] Sharma K, Lamichhane P, Sharma B, Sharma B. Sonographic measurement of spleen in relation to age: A prospective study among adult Nepalese people in Western Nepal. Journal of Gandaki Medical College-Nepal. 2017;**10**(1):11-16

[34] Chakraborti S, Saha N, Debbarma B, Das S, Leishram D. Normal spleen length by ultrasonography in adults of Tripura. Journal of Dental and Medical Sciences. 2016;**1**:55-60

[35] Arora N, Sharma P, Sahai A, Singh R. Sonographic measurements of the spleen in relation to age; a prospective study in north Indian adults. Journal of Anatomical Society of India. 2010;**59**(2):177-181

[36] Mittal R, Chowdhary D. A pilot study of the normal measurements of the liver and spleen by ultrasonography in the Rajasthani population. Journal of Clinical and Diagnostic Research. 2010;**4**(4):2733-2736

[37] Badran DH, Kalbouneh HM, Al-Hadidi MT, Shatarat AT, Tarawneh ES, Hadidy AM, et al. Ultrasonographic assessment of splenic volume and its correlation with body parameters in a Jordanian population. Saudi Medical Journal. 2015;**36**(8):967

[38] Chow KU, Luxembourg B, Seifried E, Bonig H. Spleen size is significantly influenced by body height and sex: Establishment of normal values for spleen size at US with a cohort of 1200 healthy individuals. Radiology. 2015;**279**(1):306-313

[39] Gul S, Itoo MS, Jahangir M, Kamal Y. Sonologic Assessment of Dimensions of Spleen in Normal Adult Kashmiri Population and their Correlation with Weight and Height. Autopsies Forensic Medicine and Anatomy Research. 2014;**2**:63-69

[40] Paul L, Talhar S, Sontakke B, Shende M, Waghmare J. Relation between Renal Length and Renal Volume with Patient's BMI: A Critical Appraisal. Anatomy & Physiology. 2016;**6**(246):1-7

[41] De Odorico I, Spaulding KA, Pretorius DH, Lev-Toaff AS, Bailey TB, Nelson TR. Normal splenic volumes estimated using three-dimensional ultrasonography. Journal of Ultrasound in Medicine. 1999;**18**(3):231-236

[42] Chakraborti S, Saha N, Debbarma B, Das S, Leishram D. Normal spleen length by ultrasonography in adults of Tripura. IOSR Journal of Dental and Medical Sciences. 2016;**15**(1):55-60

[43] Okuma H, Gonoi W, Ishida M, Shirota G, Kanno S, Shintani Y, et al. Comparison of volume and attenuation of the spleen between postmortem and antemortem computed tomography. International Journal of Legal Medicine. 2016;**130**(4):1081-1087

[44] Palmiere C, Tettamanti C, Scarpelli MP, Tse R. The forensic spleen: Morphological, radiological, and toxicological investigations. Forensic Science International. 2018;**291**:94-99

[45] Çeliktas M, Özandaç S, Göker P, Bozkir MG. Sonographic determination of normal spleen size in Turkish adults. International Journal of Morphology. 2015;**33**(4):1401-1405

[46] Sonmez G, Ozturk E, Basekim CC, Mutlu H, Kilic S, Onem Y, et al. Effects of altitude on spleen volume: Sonographic assessment. Journal of Clinical Ultrasound. 2007;**35**(4):182-185

[47] Purdy GM, James MA, Rees JL, Ondrus P, Keess JL, Day TA, et al. Spleen reactivity during incremental ascent to altitude. Journal of Applied Physiology. 2019;**126**(1):152-159

[48] Shephard RJ. Responses of the human spleen to exercise. Journal of Sports Sciences. 2016;**34**(10):929-936

[49] Murphy WG. The sex difference in haemoglobin levels in adults—Mechanisms, causes, and consequences. Blood Reviews. 2014;**28**(2):41-47

[50] Siddiqui MA, Ali A, Serhan O. Estimation of standard splenic volume in Saudi Arabian adult population: Using 3D reconstruction of Abdominal CT scan Images. Journal of Morphological Sciences. 2015; **32**(04):227-230

[51] Ehimwenma O, Tagbo MT. Determination of normal dimension of the spleen by ultrasound in an endemic tropical environment. Nigerian Medical Journal: Journal of the Nigeria Medical Association. 2011;**52**(3):198

[52] Ahmed OF, Assessment of normal hepatosplenic span using ultrasound in Egyptian population. Natural Science. 2017;**15**(8):215-219

[53] Galal OM. The nutrition transition in Egypt: Obesity, undernutrition and the food consumption context. Public Health Nutrition. 2002;**5**(1a):141-148

[54] Himamoni D, Das T, Talukdar K. Age related histological changes of human spleen. IJHRMLP. 2016; **3**(1):59-61

[55] Turner VM, Mabbott NA. Influence of ageing on the microarchitecture of the spleen and lymph nodes. Biogerontology. 2017;**18**(5):723-738

[56] Alex L, Rajan ML, Xavier B, Jacob P, Rani KD, Lakshmi GV. Microscopic study of human spleen in different age groups. International Journal of Research in Medical Sciences. 2015;**3**(7):1701-1706

[57] Estephan MF, Al-Saadi WI, Funjan MM. Possible anthropometric explanation of age-related changes in splenic volume in a sample of healthy Iraqi individuals using ultrasonography Iraqi Journal of Medical Sciences. 2012;**10**(4):312-320

[58] Mustapha Z, Tahir A, Tukur M, Bukar M, Lee W-K. Sonographic determination of normal spleen size in an adult African population. European Journal of Radiology. 2010;**75**(1): e133-e1e5

[59] Yousef M. Local reference of splenic volume in healthy sudanese subjects sonographically. Journal of Biomedical Engineering and Medical Imaging. 2018;**5**(4):30

Chapter 2

Ultrasound of the Pediatric Gastrointestinal Emergencies

Ercan Ayaz

Abstract

With recent technologies, ultrasound has become an extremely useful imaging modality for evaluating children with acute abdominal symptoms. Higher frequency transducers can be used in children than in adults, owing to their small body size, the presence of less fat tissue in the abdominal wall and peritoneal cavity leading to higher resolution than computed tomography in many circumstances without exposure to ionizing radiation. Real-time ultrasound imaging provides information about motion such as peristalsis, and newly developed harmonic imaging enables improved resolution with decreased artifacts. Beyond gray-scale ultrasound, color Doppler ultrasound provides information on vascularity which increases in inflammatory processes. Point-of-care examination includes ability to focus on the symptomatic area of the patient while performing real-time ultrasound imaging. Ultrasound is sufficient for the diagnosis of several gastrointestinal diseases that cause acute abdominal pain in pediatric patients helping to an accurate patient management in the emergency settings. Common gastrointestinal indications for abdominal ultrasound in children are hypertrophic pyloric stenosis, acute appendicitis, intussusception, inflammatory bowel disease, malrotation, midgut volvulus, hernia, and necrotizing enterocolitis. In this chapter, typical sonographic findings of aforementioned diseases, and possible differential diagnoses were discussed.

Keywords: Acute appendicitis, intussusception, inguinal hernia, necrotizing enterocolitis, hypertrophic pyloric stenosis, inflammatory bowel disease

1. Introduction

Non-traumatic acute gastrointestinal (GI) disorders are common causes of presentation in the pediatric emergency department. Children have wide range of potential diagnosis, different from adults including congenital and acquired lesions. The causes of acute abdomen vary according to ages of the children. Since children are unable to give reliable history, have atypical presentations and accompanying extra-abdominal manifestations; evaluation and establishing the correct diagnosis is challenging.

Traditionally, pediatric abdominal ultrasound (US) examination focuses exclusively on parenchymal organs, putting less interest on the gastrointestinal tract [1]. However, recent US technologies and new transducers are able to perform a detailed examination with great contrast resolution of each section of the digestive system in pediatric age because of their smaller body size and less impaired by gas content and adipose tissues. The other well-known advantages of US, particularly its lack of ionizing radiation, easy access, low-cost and without need of patient preparation, makes this imaging modality an ideal one for the evaluation of pediatric population in the emergency settings. Currently in many places, US is the first line of imaging over computed tomography (CT) and radiography for patients with acute abdominal pain. The main role of diagnostic imaging with US and color Doppler in the emergency is to determine whether the acute abdomen is due to a surgically or medically treatable disease, even though the exact pathology has not been diagnosed.

This chapter presents the basic aspects of US for evaluating the pediatric GI tract, including techniques, equipment, patient preparation and the anatomy. Then indications and sonographic findings of frequently encountered acute non-traumatic GI diseases in neonates, infants and children are highlighted with some exemplary cases. Acute traumatic GI tract injuries, oncologic emergencies, acute abdomen due to hepatobiliary or urogenital diseases are beyond the scope of this chapter.

2. Ultrasound technique and appropriate equipment

New generation ultrasound equipment including the wide spectrum frequency probes provides high quality images of the gastrointestinal system, adjacent mesentery and related structures. Children's small body habitus and the presence of less fat tissue in the abdominal wall enable examination with high frequency transducers. Therefore US is increasingly used as the initial and follow-up study for investigating gastrointestinal tract pathologies in children and it is sufficient for the radiological diagnosis in majority of cases.

The contrast resolution of an US probe is dependent on the frequency, the velocity of sound in tissue and the number of cycles in the US pulse [2]. Depending on the age and size of the patient, a large convex-array (1–5 MHz) or smaller convex-array transducer (5–8 MHz) is a good option for beginning the examination for overview of the entire abdomen [3]. Following initial overview, a detailed analysis of the bowel wall and adjacent structures should be evaluated with a high frequency (10–18 MHz) linear-array transducer [1]. Tissue harmonic imaging is newly developed imaging software to increase resolution of the superficial parts of the field-of-view. It should be used to improve the delineation of bowel wall layers [2]. While evaluating anxious children in the acute setting, dynamic range should be lowered and the number of foci should be reduced to increase frame rate [4]. To demonstrate peristalsis, normal or abnormal motility, and motion of air bubbles in perforation or necrotizing enterocolitis; extended field-of-view can be helpful and cine clips should be recorded [5].

Doppler US evaluation is essential in GI system imaging, especially when looking at inflammatory diseases or neoplastic conditions. Doppler should be performed with a low wall filter and pulse repetition frequency should be adjusted as low as possible to prevent aliasing [6]. Power Doppler is a good method to overcome motion artifact in uncooperative children. As there are modern equipment and software, newer vascular imaging techniques, such as B-flow and superb microvascular imaging are brought into use by different vendors which are able to assess smaller vessels in the bowel wall [4].

US elastography is an emerging US technique to assess the stiffness of a tissue [5]. There are some studies in the literature regarding the usage of elastography for GI tract diseases, particularly in inflammatory conditions [7, 8]. The bowel is a hollow viscus with a lumen containing gas and fecal contents. The anatomy of the bowel is not ideal for US elastography as solid organs (e.g. liver or kidney). However, bowel wall thickening due to inflammation or tumor often reduces motility and luminal contents that enable to perform US elastography more reliable [2]. Some studies suggest using US elastography in inflammatory bowel disease to differentiate inflammatory and fibrotic stenosis [9, 10].

Contrast enhanced US (CEUS) can be used to evaluate bowel wall vascularity and perfusion in real time [5]. It is performed after the intravenous injection of microbubbles that resonate and give rise to more intensely reflected signals [2]. Enhancement pattern, contrast quantification at peak intensity and dynamic contrast enhancement can be analyzed with CEUS [11, 12]. Enhancement pattern following bolus injection is used as a qualitative parameter. For example, patients with absent bowel wall enhancement can be separated from those with detected enhancement [2]. It can also be used in patients with complicated GI disorders when trying to differentiate a phlegmon from an abscess [13].

US examination of GI system must involve a systematic approach. While evaluating large bowel, the transducer is applied to the right iliac fossa to identify the cecum. Afterwards, colon can be followed through the ascending colon, transverse colon, descending colon, sigmoid colon and finally the rectum. Since the rectum is visualized behind the bladder, filled bladder is better to evaluate rectum and sigmoid colon. Longitudinal placement of the transducer is often better to identify the haustrations of colon segments [2]. The examination of the small intestine begins with the identification of ileocecal valve and the terminal ileum at the right iliac fossa. The examiner should identify the appendix, often inferior to the terminal ileum and follow the ileum as far as possible. Tracking the whole small bowel is generally not possible, therefore the abdomen should be scanned cranially and caudally parallel scans covering the whole abdominal area. The scanning approach may differ according to clinical scenario. For surgical disorders or trauma, a faster and a targeted approach are preferred, whereas for general and nonspecific complaints, more detailed examination can be performed.

Graded compression is a simple, essential and effective technique to push away gas filled bowel segments or intraabdominal fat [3, 4]. It decreases the distance between the transducer and target organ and enables to reach deeper with high frequency transducers. Although it was introduced for the diagnosis of acute appendicitis by Puylaert [14], now it has been performed for detection of bowel thickening and compressibility, and for specific diseases such as diverticulitis and colonic polyps [15, 16].

3. Patient preparation and clinical indications

As a general principle, no preparation of the patient is required to perform gastrointestinal US, particularly in the emergency setting. However, to decrease the amount of food and gas in the gut, and to examine the gallbladder and biliary tree, a fasting period of 3 hours in newborn and 5 hours in children is recommended [1]. Physical activity also reduces the splanchnic flow, therefore patients should avoid from extensive activity before the examination [2]. Since the cold gel is one of the major complaints of children, gel warmer to warm the coupling gel can be used. If the infants or neonates are anxious and reluctant to be scanned; examiner can sit them on their mother's lap, get her lie down on the couch along with the child.

For stomach and pyloric examination, oral fluid intake or fluid ingestion via nasogastric tube is useful [4]. The distention of colon with anechoic fluid (water) ingestion, or with oral administration of hyperosmotic solutions allows the detailed examination of the haustration of colonic wall and adjacent structure [2]. The scanning of small intestine following the ingestion of iso-osmolar polyethylene glycol (PEG) solution is called US enterography or small intestine contrast US (SICUS).

Since the PEG solution is non-absorbable in the small bowel, retained fluid distends the intestine and induces the wall contractility. The PEG solution moves distally and distends whole loops of the entire small bowel. Following PEG ingestion, small bowel lumen diameter > 30 mm and wall thickness > 3 mm is abnormal [17].

Before beginning a US examination, examiner should be familiar with the abdominal symptoms, clinical presentations and laboratory findings of acute GI diseases. The most common presentations are pain, vomiting, diarrhea, fever, hematochezia and melena. Although some diseases have peculiar clinical findings, majority of cases have non-specific symptoms and clinical appearances [3]. US is generally suggested as the first line imaging modality in children with acute abdomen. Most common indications for gastrointestinal US in children are acute appendicitis, intussusception, hernia, hypertrophic pyloric stenosis, inflammatory bowel disease, and volvulus. Further indications involve necrotizing enterocolitis, duplication cysts, malrotation of the bowel [4]. Also US is widely performed for the disease of other intraabdominal structures such as mesenteric lymphadenitis, lymphoid hyperplasia of the appendix, infectious enterocolitis, omental infarct, epiploic appendagitis, specific inflammations such as tuberculosis, colitis with hemolytic uraemic syndrome and Henoch-Schönlein purpura [4]. The recent COVID-19 pandemic associated multisystem inflammatory syndrome in children (MIS-C) can also manifest with gastrointestinal system dysfunction which has been also a novel US indication since 2020 [18].

4. Challenges of GI ultrasound

Major challenges of US is based on its operator-dependency and reproducibility [5]. The European Federation of Societies for Ultrasound in Medicine and Biology (EFSUMB) suggests to set standards of training and education curriculum for GI system US to provide high quality performance in clinical practice [2]. According to EFSUMB recommendations; the operator should be able to recognize the normal anatomy of small intestine and large bowel initially. Following recognizing normal appearance of normal GI tract, the investigator should be able to perform a complete scanning of the gut; evaluation for focal or diffuse diseases, the presence of diverticular disease and its complications (perforation and obstruction), the peritoneal cavity, the mesentery, and the omentum for the inflammatory, infectious or malignant diseases [2].

There are other challenging factors related to the patient such as noncollaboration, obesity and interposition of large amount of gas [5]. Particularly retroperitoneal, paraaortic and retroduodenal areas are often danger zones that are not well delineated on US. If the graded compression technique is ineffective to eliminate gas interposition and US findings are unremarkable; intravenous contrast enhanced CT should be performed in patients with acute abdominal pain, especially if there is suspicion of gut perforation.

5. Normal anatomy

While examining normal anatomy of GI structures; position, size, wall thickness and stratification should be evaluated. Many GI disorders appear as bowel wall thickening but normal bowel wall thickness may vary depending on peristalsis and the degree of distention [3]. Recent studies with high frequency transducers suggest that both normal small and large bowel wall thickness should be <2 mm when distended [19]. The exceptions are the pylor/duodenal bulbus and rectum wall which should be < 3 mm and < 4 mm respectively [20]. If the measurements were made from collapsed bowel wall, it should be reported since the wall of collapsed bowel is shown as thicker [2].

When examined with high frequency transducers, five sonographic layers of the bowel wall can be seen. When imaging the anterior wall (closer to transducer); the innermost echogenic layer is called as the mucosa-lumen interface which is not a part of actual GI wall. The second hypoechoic layer correspond to the deep mucosa, the third hyperechoic layer is submucosa which is most prominent in the colon [3]. The muscularis propria is the hypoechoic fourth layer which is most pronounced in the stomach. The outermost hyperechoic layer is the interface between muscularis and serosa. As the interface are hyperechoic and located distal to the real tissue, correspondence of histology and US layers are slightly different in the dorsal wall [2]. Therefore, evaluation of the layers should be made from the anterior bowel wall in diffuse inflammatory diseases. Bowel wall thickness measurement should be made perpendicular to the wall from innermost to the outermost echogenic layers [2].

The small intestine has three segments. The duodenum passes into the jejunum at the ligament of Treitz located in the left upper quadrant. The jejunum is often located in the left upper quadrant and usually collapsed with prominent folds, also known as valvula conniventes. They decrease and shorten from jejunum to ileum and best demonstrated at the fluid filled loops [2]. The ileum is located at the right lower quadrant and frequently involves fluid in normal patients. Sometimes cecum may be located intraperitoneal in variable positions even at the left lower quadrant of abdomen. The cecum and ileocecal valve is important landmarks to identify appendix which is usually below to the ileocecal valve. Although appendix is typically seen over the iliopsoas muscle medial to the cecum, lateral elevation or retrocecal course are not infrequent [2]. The normal appendix can be visualized in about 70% of healthy children with graded compression and it may increase depending on the experience of examiner and the resolution of transducer [21].

6. Acute appendicitis

Acute appendicitis accounts for 80% of all abdominal surgical emergencies in pediatric population [22]. It is most frequently seen in second decade and is rare in children under two years of age, probably due to the funnel shape of appendix in infancy, which reduces the possibility of obstruction [23, 24]. Possible predisposing factors include lymphoid hyperplasia (due to past viral infection), dehydration, and low dietary intake of fiber [24]. Although the typical clinical presentation is acute onset of abdominal pain that may occur in the periumbilical area, radiating to the right lower quadrant, one-third of children have atypical clinical findings and symptoms, especially younger ones [23]. Other clinical signs are; fever, elevated acute phase reactants, nausea, vomiting and leg pain. Diarrhea is not present unless there is perforation and peritonitis, more frequently occurs in young children and confused with gastroenteritis [24]. Following clinical assessment and laboratory findings, imaging is the third component while evaluating the patients with suspected appendicitis. The routine US examination in suspected appendicitis reduces the negative appendectomies 50% and decreases the surgical complications and costs [25].

In patients with localized pain, transducer is applied to the point of maximum tenderness or pain. Self-localization facilitates the scanning, especially in patients with an aberrantly located appendix, and reduces the time of examination. If the patient cannot localize the pain or uncooperative; systematic evaluation starts in transvers plane to identify ascending colon. Lowermost part of the ascending colon is the cecal pole and medial to the cecum ileocecal valve can be demonstrated. The most common origin of the appendix is 2–3 cm below to the ileocecal valve [26]. Pressure is gradually increased to displace gas and fecal materials in the cecal lumen to adduct appendix to the transducer. In obese children, a left oblique body position or an upward graded compression technique may be useful to displace the fat tissue of the abdominal wall [27]. Anatomical variations require a systematic approach to evaluate appendix and experience plays an important role in examination. There are several US features to distinguish between normal and inflamed appendix which are valid for both children and adults (**Table 1**) [25, 26, 28, 29].

The inflamed appendix is shown as a fluid-filled non-compressible distended aperistaltic tubular structure with a blind end (**Figure 1**). In the axial plane, it has a target appearance with thickened echogenic mucosal interface and hypoechoic muscular wall. Appearance of an appendicolith, which is an echogenic focus with a posterior acoustic shadowing, is supportive finding for the diagnosis (**Figure 1C**) [23]. However, intraluminal air is also echogenic and can mimic appendicolith (**Figure 1D**). A heterogeneous mass around appendix representing phlegmon, and a walled-off fluid collection representing abscess are often the signs of complicated appendicitis and perforation [23]. Complicated appendicitis can occur either as a gangrenous appendicitis (focal or diffuse necrosis of the wall) or as a perforation. There is continuous transition from phlegmonous uncomplicated to gangrenous appendicitis during the disease course. The most important indicator of gangrenous appendicitis is the loss of normal hyperechoic mucosa-lumen interface [30]. Other ancillary finding is the lack of vascularity on color Doppler. The rate of perforation following acute appendicitis is around 60% for a 3-year-old child, 50% for a 5-year-old child, and this incidence reduces with increasing age, because of limited ability to communicate and define complaints in little ones [31]. Moreover, small children are more prone to peritonitis and abscess formation, rather than phlegmon, following perforation due to underdeveloped omentum which confines purulent material [24].

Non-visualization of the appendix is an important problem while evaluating appendicitis. The major reason for false-negative scanning is inexperience examiner in GI US. Other challenging situations are retrocecal or pelvic position of appendix, thick abdominal fat tissue in very obese patients, or focal appendicitis confined to distal tip that account for 5% of cases [25]. Thus, the entire appendix should be delineated clearly [32]. In perforated appendicitis, an abscess may be misinterpreted as a gas-containing bowel loop. In these cases, indirect signs of appendicitis should be scrutinized around cecum [33].

Primary US findings of acute appendicitis	Secondary US findings of acute appendicitis (adjacent structures)
Maximum outer diameter > 6 (6–8 mm indicates borderzone)	Hyperechoic periappendiceal fat tissue
Maximum tenderness over the thickened appendix	Complex fluid collection (pericecal abscess)
Incompressibility of the inflamed appendix	Mesenteric / pericecal lymphadenopathy
Appendicolith (fecalith) within the appendix lumen	Periappendiceal reactive fluid
Hypervascularity in color Doppler in uncomplicated cases	
Loss of stratification and normal appearance of appendix wall in gangrenous appendicitis	

Table 1.
Primary and secondary sonographic features of acute appendicitis.

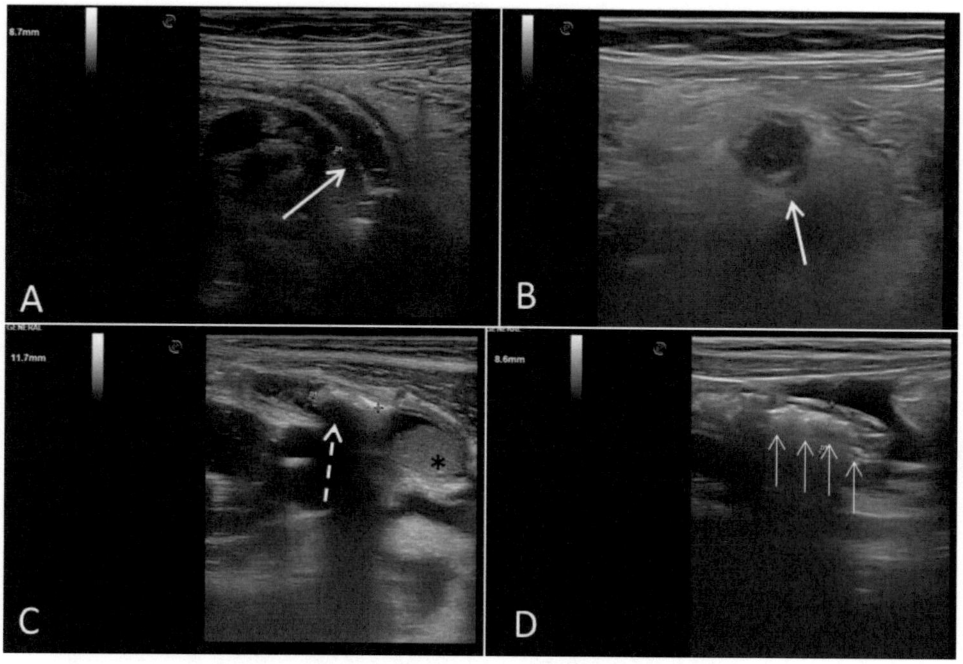

Figure 1.
Three different cases with acute appendicitis. Ultrasound images of an 8-year-old boy demonstrate longitudinal (A) and transverse (B) section of inflamed appendix (arrow) with a diameter of 8.7 mm, and hyperechoic inflamed periappendiceal fat tissue. Ultrasound image of a 9-year-old boy (C) shows appendicolith (dashed arrow) within the appendix lumen, fluid level (asterisk) and dilatation distal to the obstruction. Ultrasound image of a 5-year-old girl (D) demonstrates inflamed appendix with a diameter of 8.6 mm and periappendiceal reactive fluid. Despite the inflammation, lumen is filled with air seen as echogenicity with dirty posterior shadow (thin arrows).

Recent publications confirm the mild forms of appendicitis which is spontaneously resolved under antibiotic therapy without need for surgery [34]. Unfortunately, there are not any reliable criteria to differentiate mild courses on US that probably not require surgery [25]. Other pitfalls that lead to a false-positive diagnosis of acute appendicitis are; incorrect identification of the terminal ileum as inflamed appendix, Meckel's diverticulitis, cecal diverticulitis, dilated Fallopian tube or gonadal vein thrombosis [25]. Contrarily, appendiceal thickening can occur by other conditions such as Crohn's disease, infectious enterocolitis, peritonitis, ascites and appendiceal tumors such as mucocele, cystadenoma or carcinoid [25].

Over the last decades, the sensitivity of US for the diagnosis of appendicitis has reached to 95%, with specificity above 90% [23, 35, 36]. The accuracy of US is currently equivalent to CT and magnetic resonance imaging (MRI), even more accurate particularly in small children with less intraabdominal fat tissue. Point-of-care ultrasonography (POCUS) is increasingly done by emergency physicians for the diagnosis of appendicitis, but US is a highly operator dependent tool that requires experience and sufficient equipment. Consequently, adequate equipment, structured training program and quality control should be provided before clinical application. Consistent preoperative use of US for right lower quadrant pain can decrease the additional CT/MRI examinations to a low fraction [35, 37]. When initial US is inconclusive, second US following an observation period, or an additional MRI or CT examination can be considered. In children, MRI should be performed if possible to support the ALARA (radiation as low as reasonably achievable) principle. Some guidelines recommend several scoring systems for US to diagnose acute appendicitis [38]. Since these scoring systems roughly estimate the likelihood and do not prove appendicitis, they are not obligatory to use in routine practice [25].

7. Hypertrophic pyloric stenosis

Hypertrophic pyloric stenosis (HPS) is the most common cause of surgery in vomiting infants due to the failure of relaxation of the pyloric sphincter of stomach [39]. The disease usually appears between 2nd and 12th week of life and commonly affects white males [2, 39]. The typical complaint is non-bilious, projecting vomiting by a previously healthy infant after feeding. HPS is not an actual emergency unless severe dehydration or excessive electrolyte loss occur. HPS can be palpated as a pyloric mass in the epigastrium on physical examination (olive sign) [22]. Preoperative US is the gold standard radiologic modality for the diagnosis of HPS with sensitivity, specificity and accuracy of approximately 100% if adequate equipment is provided [40].

The US scanning begins with placing the baby in a supine or right lateral decubitus position. A high-frequency (10–18 MHz), linear-array transducer should be applied from sub-xiphoid area to the right paramedian area to search for pylorus [1]. If adequate fluid is not present in the stomach, breast feeding or oral sugar contained water can be given in order to displace the air in the stomach and to see the passage of the fluid [41]. Normal position of the pylorus can be demonstrated between the liver and the head of the pancreas, medial to the gallbladder. If abundant air present in the gastric antrum, the patient should be moved into the right lateral decubitus position, to displace air into the fundus and to move pylorus anteriorly [3]. To confirm the HPS, pyloric canal length and thickness of the pyloric muscle should be measured [1]. Pyloric muscle thickness > 3 mm, canal length > 17 mm, and antero-posterior diameter of pylorus >12 mm confirm the diagnosis of HPS with high accuracy (**Figure 2**) [1, 3, 22]. By the way, pylorus is a dynamic structure and muscle thickness may change due to peristalsis during a real-time US examination. Therefore, imaging for a sufficient time is needed to exclude pylorospasm from HPS, which is a transient phenomenon [41]. Other ancillary findings to diagnose HPS are the prolapsed mucosa into the gastric antrum (antral nipple or cervix sign) and trapped fluid within the crevices of mucosa. The main reason of false-negative result is the overdistention of stomach that moves antra-pyloric canal posteriorly [3]. To overcome this issue, gastric content can be aspirated via nasogastric or orogastric tube.

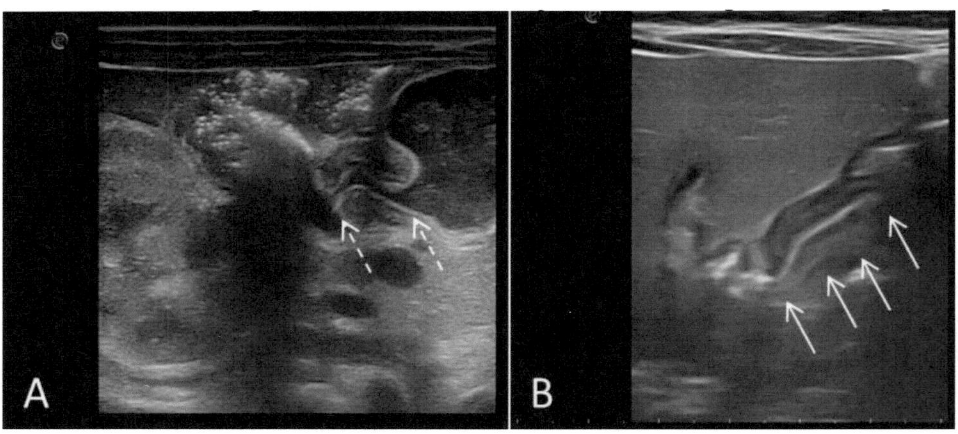

Figure 2.
(A) Normal appearance of pylor in a 25-day-old baby and (B) hypertrophic pyloric stenosis in a 30-day-old boy. Hypertrophic pylor (arrows) is thicker and longer than normal (dashed arrows) that does not permit the passage of gastric content into the duodenum.

8. Intussusception

Intussusception is the penetration of the bowel segment, either the small intestine or colon, into the distal lumen and propulsion as luminal content. It is the most common etiology of small bowel obstruction in infants, with a reported incidence of 56 cases per 100,000 hospitalizations per year in the United States [24]. More than 90% of cases present in the first two years after birth and peak age between 3 and 9 months [1, 3, 22]. Depending on the localization, there are two subtypes; ileo-cecal (or ileocolic) comprises 90% of cases and ileo-ileal occurs in about 10% [42]. The most common symptoms are recurrent abdominal pain, vomiting and currant jelly stool. Additionally, previous episodes of infection in the upper respiratory tract or gastroenteritis may occur in the patient's clinical history. Most common localization of ileocecal intussusception is the subhepatic region, followed by upper abdominal midline and left upper quadrant [3]. It consists of three bowel segments; the inner prolapsing and returning limbs of the bowel are terminal ileum (called as intussusceptum) and attached mesentery and lymph nodes is dragged between these limbs [3, 39]. Outermost bowel receiving intussusceptum is the colon (called as intussuscipiens). Due to the compromised vascular supply, the thickest ileal segment is the returning limb of the ileum [3].

The diagnostic accuracy of US have verified with the several studies with a sensitivity of 97–100% and a specificity of 88–100% [24]. Thus, US has become as the primary modality of choice, replacing the contrast enema, in patients with suspected intussusception. Transverse section of intussusception appears as an oval or round mass with concentric rings and hypoechoic rim, described as 'doughnut' or 'target' configuration on US [1]. The crescentic shaped, hyperechoic, mesenteric fat can be seen in the center of the mass (called as 'the crescent in doughnut sign') (**Figure 3A** and **B**). The longitudinal appearance of intussusception is called as 'pseudo-kidney' or 'sandwich' sign (**Figure 3C**). On color Doppler US, double rings sign between the layers can be seen (**Figure 3B**) and absence of blood flow may indicate ischemia or irreducibility [22]. US can also be performed safely and accurately to monitor the hydrostatic reduction. Successful hydrostatic reduction rates are approximately 80% with a very few complication rates (2.7%to 4.26%) [24]. Some findings on US are useful to predict the success of enema or hydrostatic reduction such as; reduced vascular flow, thickened outer wall (>10 mm), trapped fluid and/or large (>1 cm short axis) lymph nodes within the intussusceptum [1, 3]. The appearance of intramural or subserosal air,

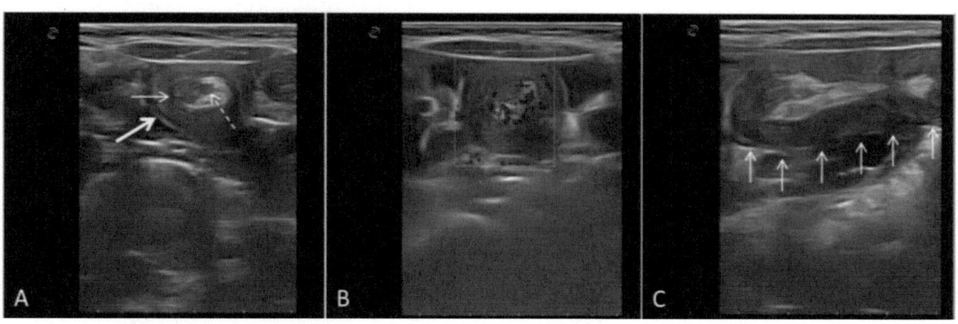

Figure 3.
A 5-month-old boy with intussusception. (A) Transverse section demonstrates "target sign" composed of intussusceptum (thin arrow), intussuscipiens (thick arrow) and a lymph node (dashed arrow) within the trapped mesenteric fat tissue. (B) Doppler shows swirling of arteries and veins within intussusception. (C) Longitudinal section shows typical "sandwich" or "pseudokidney" sign (arrows).

manifested as echogenic foci, indicates the risk of necrosis and perforation, for those enema/hydrostatic reduction is contraindicated [1].

The US can identify pathologic lead points in approximately two third of cases, particularly in older age group [43]. Similarly pathologic lead points may occur in younger than expected age group as < 3 months of age [24]. Common lead points are; Meckel's diverticulum, duplication cyst, lymphoma or polyp. Cystic fibrosis, Henoch-Schonlein purpura, or polyposis syndrome may cause recurrent intussusceptions. Lead points or underlying disease should be searched elaborately in a patient with unusual age, abnormal localization of intussusception, recurrent disease and long duration of symptoms [3].

Small bowel intussusception comprises 10% of cases and is usually transient and asymptomatic. Common locations are the periumbilical area, left upper or lower quadrant of the abdomen. Most cases are due to small bowel hyperperistalsis. They are usually smaller than ileocecal intussusception (<1 cm diameter) and involve shorter bowel segment. If small bowel intussusception is persistent and symptomatic or involving longer segment (>3.5 cm), the patient should be scrutinized carefully to identify pathological lead point [3].

9. Intestinal malrotation and volvulus

Intestinal malrotaton is not an infrequent phenomenon with a prevalence of 0,2–0,5% of live births. While the most patients are asymptomatic, 3–8% of malrotated bowel is symptomatic in the first year of life with bilious vomiting, pain and malabsorption [1]. The normal midgut rotates 270^0 counterclockwise in utero around the axis of superior mesenteric artery (SMA). Incomplete rotation of bowel during fetal period results in short mesenteric root, abnormal positioning of duodeno-jejunal junction and ileocecal valve and close proximity of duodenum and cecum [3]. Twisting of malrotated small bowel around its mesentery may cause obstruction and volvulus, an emergent situation that requires prompt surgical intervention [44].

The well-known sonographic finding of intestinal malrotation is the inversion of the SMA and superior mesenteric vein (SMV). Patients should be lay supine while US evaluation and transducer applied at the upper midline to recognize SMA at its point of origin on the abdominal aorta [1]. SMV can also be identified tracing from the main portal vein to the midline after giving branch of splenic vein. Normally, the SMV is found on the right side or anterior to the SMA. If SMV located ventrally or left to the SMA, it is an abnormal location, which raises suspicion but do not always indicate malrotation [3]. For evaluating duodenum and to see the passage or beak sign of acute volvulus, oral water instillation may be useful. In suspected malrotation patients, when US findings are abnormal or inconclusive, an upper GI study should be performed, as a gold standard, to confirm the diagnosis [45].

Midgut volvulus is a fatal complication of malrotation, and 90% of cases occur in the first year of life, even %75 of cases occur in the first month. The typical sonographic feature of volvulus is the 'whirlpool sign', which is the swirling of SMV and its tributaries around the SMA in clockwise direction, best appreciated on color Doppler. Associated US findings of malrotation are proximal duodenal dilatation with distal tapering, duodenal wall thickening (> 2 mm), fixed midline bowel, intraabdominal free fluid, dilatation of the distal SMV and increased resistive index on SMA [3, 39].

Off-midline scanning due to inappropriate position of the transducer may demonstrate SMV and SMA as an abnormal relation which is the most common cause of the false-positive diagnosis of malrotation. Another reason for false-positive diagnosis is the 'whirlpool' sign occurs due to normal counterclockwise rotation. False-negative diagnosis may also be observed due to severe abdominal distension, abdominal guarding, abundant bowel gas, and/or an inexperienced operator. If there is strong clinical suspicion, an emergency upper GI study should be performed to clarify the diagnosis [3].

10. Necrotizing enterocolitis

Necrotizing enterocolitis (NEC) is one of the most common and lethal gastrointestinal emergencies of neonates, usually affecting the terminal ileum and ascending colon [22]. Although it affects primarily preterm babies, NEC can also be seen in term infants. The clinical presentation ranges from feeding intolerance, abdominal distention, emesis, diarrhea, rectal bleeding to more severe systemic findings including respiratory failure and fulminant shock [41]. Bowel necrosis occurs in NEC without any precise cause, which compromises the mucosal integrity [6]. Pathogenic organisms become dominant in the gut flora, leading to the pneumatosis intestinalis, which subsequently leads to portal venous gas and consequently leads to perforation and pneumoperitoneum. While the disease progresses, both early and late clinical signs and laboratory tests are often non-specific for diagnosis of NEC, therefore imaging plays crucial role for accurate diagnosis.

Radiographs are still primary modality of choice for evaluation of neonates suspected of having NEC [46]. Plain abdominal radiographs demonstrate pneumatosis, increased thickness of bowel wall, free intraperitoneal air and portal venous air [22, 46]. The role of US has been increasingly appreciated, owing to its higher sensitivity than plain films in the detection of early changes such as wall thickening, intestinal pneumatosis, portal venous air and disturbed bowel wall perfusion on color Doppler [5, 46]. Recent publications stated that diagnostic performance of US for detecting NEC is accurate with sensitivity of 100% and specificity of 90%. However, role of US in the follow-up of NEC is uncertain [6].

In the early phase of the disease, US can show the bowel wall thickening due to inflammation. Whereas, bowel wall thinning (<1 mm) may occur as it becomes necrotic and progresses toward perforation [47]. Similarly, Color Doppler may display hyperemia in the early stages due to inflammation, and avascular wall in the advanced disease with bowel wall necrosis [6]. Pneumatosis intestinalis is seen as punctate or granular echogenic foci with 'dirty' posterior acoustic shadowing or linear echogenic ring within the bowel wall. The gas bubbles create twinkling artifact on color Doppler which is useful in equivocal cases. To differentiate intramural gas from intraluminal air, nondependent bowel wall should be evaluated. Moreover, true pneumatosis would not change with the motion of the patient, whereas intraluminal air is freely mobile. Placing the patient in multiple positions may be useful to observe movement of the air. For the detection of pneumatosis, US is more sensitive than plain radiography [48].

Portal venous gas manifests on US as the presence of curvilinear or punctate mobile echogenic foci within the portal venous system. It is commonly seen in the neonates after umbilical catheterization, and may occur in different neonatal diseases. Therefore, in the absence of pneumatosis intestinalis, other etiologies should be considered rather than NEC. In the case of NEC, fluid-filled dilated bowel, complex hyperechoic intraperitoneal free fluid, focal fluid collections are suggestive of perforation and have been correlated with a poor clinical outcome [47, 49]. Evaluation of bowel peristalsis by real-time examination is an important component of US in infants with suspected NEC, because necrotic or inflamed bowel segments have decreased or absent motility [6]. US may also be considered in the follow-up to decide the appropriate time to restore oral feeding and to evaluate post-enterocolitis stenosis [5].

11. Inflammatory and infectious bowel diseases

Inflammatory bowel disease (IBD) is a general term that covers a series of acute and non-acute diseases which do not require surgical treatment, ranging from self-limiting focal disorders to the debilitating and/or chronic diseases [1]. Diagnosis can be challenging due to nonspecific or atypical clinical presentation with extra-intestinal manifestations. US is useful in the diagnosis of IBD, especially in children by assessing bowel wall, peristalsis and surrounding mesentery with high-frequency transducers. Moreover, color Doppler increases the diagnostic accuracy and estimates the disease activity by showing vascularity. Presence of extra-intestinal complications such as abscess, fistula can also be evaluated with US.

While evaluating IBD, the thickening of the bowel wall can be divided into two categories according to US appearance [1]. 'Layered thickening' is shown as hyper-echoic and organized wall thickening corresponds to mucosal inflammation with indirect involvement of submucosa. Whereas 'non-layered thickening' characterized by the loss of normal structure seen as a diffuse hypoechoic thickening without any reflective echoes. Based on the thickening type and localization, possible diagnoses are presented in **Table 2**.

Crohn disease is the most common IBD that requires frequent imaging because of its extensive involvement of GI tract, and phases of exacerbations and remissions [1, 6]. It is characterized as a chronic transmural inflammation of an unknown cause and can affect any part of GI tract. In 20% of cases, the disease first becomes symptomatic during childhood [39]. Although, the role in the diagnostic algorithm is emerging, bowel US in its current form cannot replace with CT or MRI but can provide complementary information in the evaluation of disease. The diagnostic performance of US for identifying lesions of Crohn disease has sensitivity of 75–94% and specificity of 67–100% [6]. The primary imaging features of Crohn disease are bowel wall thickening and loss of stratification. Affected segments are non-compressible, hypoperistaltic and have hypoechoic wall with a minimal thickness of >3 mm [6, 39]. The hallmark of active disease is increased vascularity of thickened bowel wall segments (> 5 mm) with 88% specificity and 95% positive predictive value [49]. Moreover, SMA flow volume is higher but resistive index is lower with active disease [6]. Remarkable extramural manifestations that can be seen on US include thickened, hyperechoic mesentery ('creeping fat' sign) and enlarged mesenteric lymph nodes (**Figure 4**). Strictures, fistula, phlegmon and abscess are common complications of Crohn disease that can be depicted on US but requires further evaluation with CT or MRI. On US strictures are identified in

	Ileum involvement	Colon involvement
Layered thickening	Infectious ileitis (Campylobacter or salmonella)	Infectious colitis (E.Coli, salmonella, shigella)
	Early Crohn disease	Chronic intestinal infectious disease (CIID)
Non-layered thickening	Henoch-Schönlein Purpura	Ischemic colitis prodromal of hemolytic uremic syndrome (HUS)
	Tuberculosis ileitis	Advanced IBD (ulcerative colitis or Crohn disease)
	Protein-losing enteropathy, Celiac disease	Pseudomembranous colitis
	Advanced Crohn disease	Neutropenic colitis

Table 2.
Sonographic pattern and location of common inflammatory bowel diseases.

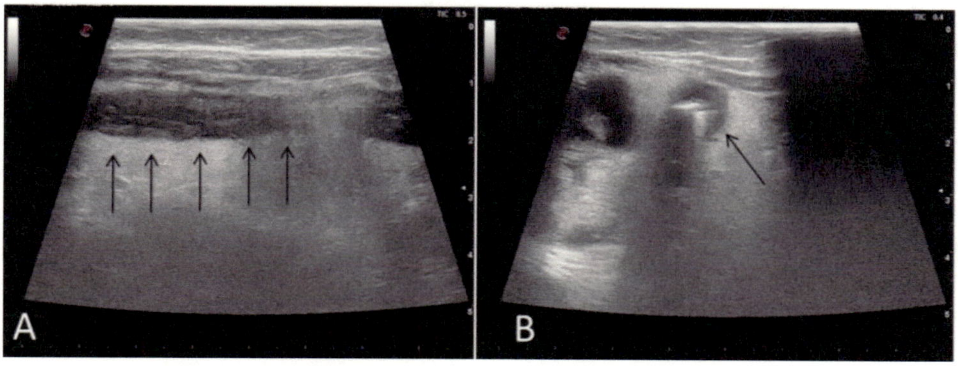

Figure 4.
An active Crohn's disease in an 11-year-old girl. Longitudinal (A) and transverse (B) section of inflamed bowel segments demonstrates layered wall thickening, increased echogenicity and prominent thickening of mesenteric fat tissue.

70–79% of cases as a narrowed bowel segment accompanying dilatation and hyperperistalsis at the proximal part [6]. Fistulas are less common in children than adults, and US is not a reliable modality to depict fistulas with the sensitivity of 31–87% in different publications [50]. An abscess can be delineated with US as an irregular thick-walled aperistaltic fluid collection including internal echoes and sometimes air. The sensitivity of US for the diagnosis of abscessranges from 83–91% [51]. An abscess may mimic a bowel loop, but bowel segments are thin-walled and peristalsis of bowel can be seen on real-time imaging.

Henoch-Schönlein Purpura (HSP) is the most common pediatric vasculitis that frequently involve GI tract [3, 39]. The pathogenesis of the disease originated from the thrombosis of small vessels, which in turn can cause ischemia of the small bowel [39]. Bowel wall thickening and edema can be seen on US in 50–60% of cases [52]. Although typical skin lesions are the hallmark of the disease, bowel wall thickening in duodenum and proximal small bowel may occur before the appearance of skin lesions. However, HSP can affect any segment of the bowel. The most common US feature is diffuse circumferential bowel wall thickening (**Figure 5**). Focal intramural hemorrhage can be revealed as a hyperechoic lesion in the mucosa or submucosa. With intramural hematoma, bowel wall thickening may increase up to 9–10 mm and multiple skip lesions can be demonstrated [3]. In HSP patients with obstructive symptoms such as vomiting or hemorrhagic stool, one or more intussusception can be seen with intramural hematoma as a lead point [53]. In the active stage of the disease, hypervascularity on color Doppler imaging may present. Other less common vasculitides involving the bowel may also occur with a variable presentation but similar findings on US.

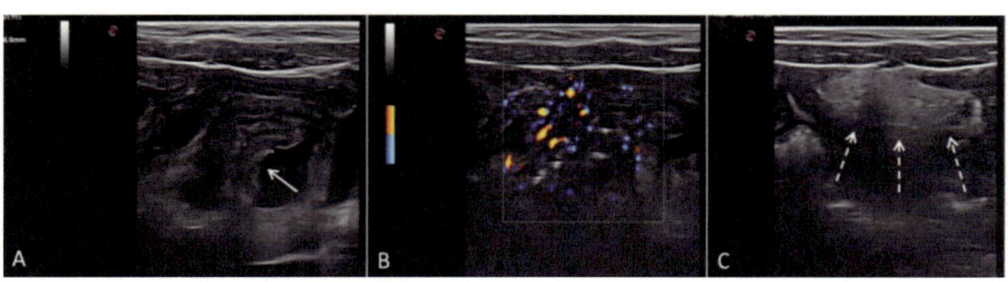

Figure 5.
An 8 year-old-girl with Henoch-Schönlein Purpura. (A) Ultrasound shows diffuse thickening of the intestinal wall (arrow). (B) Color Doppler demonstrates increased vascularity. Gray scale ultrasound from another part of abdomen (C) reveals hyperechoic mesenteric fat tissue (dashed arrows).

Bacterial enterocolitis can occur by a wide variety of pathogens, including *E. Coli*, *Salmonella*, *Shigella* and *Campylobacter*. Common location is ileocecal region and US features are similar to other inflammatory disease, such as bowel wall thickening, increased echogenicity, reactive mesenteric lymph nodes, and mild intraabdominal free fluid. Viral gastroenteritis generally does not increase the thickness of the bowel wall; however enlarged lymph nodes and free fluid may be present [41]. *Tuberculosis* may also present with bowel wall thickening along with hepatosplenomegaly, omental thickening, and typical internal echoes and septations within ascites [54]. Parasites can be revealed by US as mobile, tubular hypoechoic structures with hyperechoic rim in *Ascariasis* infection, with parallel echogenic lines representing digestive system [41].

Neutropenic colitis, also known as typhilitis, is a necrotizing inflammatory process of cecum and terminal ileum usually seen in severe neutropenic and immunocompromised patients [39]. The typical US features are asymmetric, prominent wall thickening, with decreased echogenicity and loss of layering due to transmural inflammation. Echogenic foci can be seen in the bowel wall caused by circumscriptive hemorrhages or intramural air suggestive of anaerobic infection [55]. In thyphilitis, increased wall thickness may have correlation with a worse prognosis of the disease [41].

Pseudomembranous colitis is caused by the superinfection with *C. difficile*, often following a prior course of antibiotic treatment or rarely associated with shock, uremia, heavy metal intoxication or severe cardiovascular disease. The enterotoxin of *C. difficile* leads to severe inflammatory reaction within the colon between 1 and 6 weeks after the antibiotic treatment [24]. The common clinical findings are severe generalized abdominal pain, watery diarrhea, fever, and leukocytosis. The disease causes marked mucosal thickening of the colon, even thicker than other infectious colitis. On US, apart from thick hypoechoic mucosal layer, narrowing of the gut lumen and thickened hyperechoic submucosa can be demonstrated. In the majority of patients, the hypoechoic muscularis layer, which is outer than hyperechoic submucosa, appears normal and relatively thin. Intraabdominal free fluid is present in up to 77% of cases [24].

12. Mesenteric lymphadenitis

Mesenteric lymphadenitis is a benign, self-limiting inflammatory condition that affects the mesenteric lymph nodes, more frequently pericecal ones. It may either occur as a primary inflammatory disease or may arise secondarily due to an abdominal disease. Clinically, this condition is commonly mistaken for appendicitis, since the symptoms are quite similar [22]. As the lymph node enlargement is the only finding on US, the diagnosis is made by excluding other possible etiologies of abdominal pain.

Various nomograms for normal ranges of mesenteric lymph node size have been reported and short axis of > 5 mm for lymph nodes are very common in healthy children [3]. Simanovsky et al. [56] suggested that, in the setting of normal appendix, cluster of > 3 lymph nodes with short axis of > 10 mm should be diagnosed as mesenteric lymphadenopathy. Enlarged lymph nodes are often oval and perinodal fat tissue may appear hyperechoic (**Figure 6**). A preserved fatty hilum is seen as a hyperechoic area at the center with vascular pedicle on color Doppler imaging. If the shape of enlarged lymph nodes is round rather than being oval, cortex is eccentrically thickened and there is loss of fatty hilum, neoplastic process should be suspected [3].

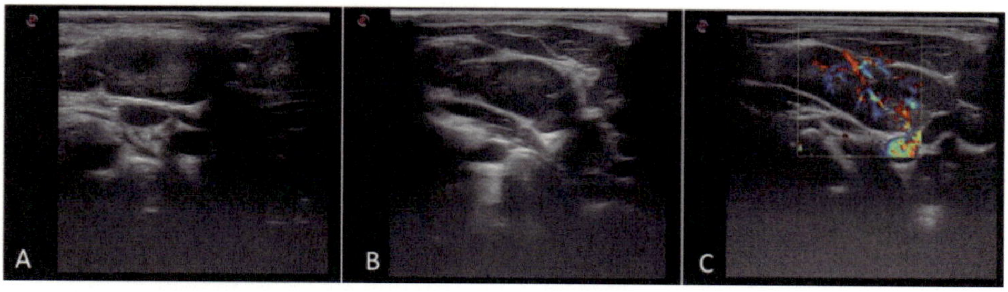

Figure 6.
Ultrasound (A,B) and color Doppler ultrasound (C) of the right lower quadrant of a 5-year-old girl diagnosed as mesenteric lymphadenitis. There are enlarged lymph nodes anterior to the iliac vessels. Color Doppler (C) demonstrates vascular supply from hilum of the lymph node.

13. Epiploic appendagitis and omental infarction

Epiploic appendagitis is the inflammation of epiploic appendages arise from the serosal surface of the large bowel. Torsion of the appendages results in venous occlusion, ischemia and inflammation [39]. Although predominantly encountered in adults, it is also described in children and should be kept in mind in the differential diagnosis of acute appendicitis because the treatment is supportive rather than surgery. Characteristic US feature is hyperechoic, fixed non-compressible oval mass-like lesion at the anti-mesenteric side of the bowel. CT is generally needed to confirm the exact diagnosis [57].

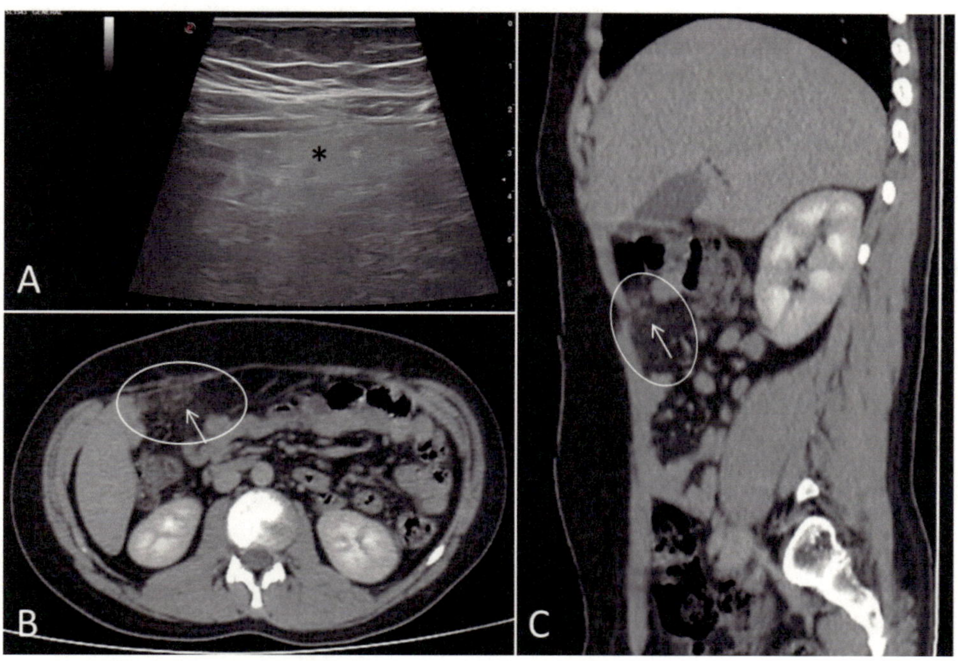

Figure 7.
Ultrasound image (A) of an 11-year-old boy demonstrates thickened hyperechoic mass (asterisk) with indistinct border beneath the anterior abdominal wall. Intravenous contrast enhanced axial CT (B) and sagittal reconstructed image (C) shows hyperdense omentum (white circles), hyperdense dot at the center of lesion (arrows). The dot can be followed on the contiguous images as a linear tortuous hyperdense structure consistent with twisted vein. Surgical removal of necrotic tissue confirmed the diagnosis of omental infarct.

Omental infarction is a rare cause of acute abdomen in children, even though 15% of all omental infarct cases occur in the pediatric population [3]. As the patients are commonly present with right-sided abdominal pain, it mimics appendicitis. However, associated nausea and vomiting is less frequent than appendicitis [24]. Predisposing factors include obesity, strenuous activity, coagulopathy and history of trauma to the affected region. The characteristic US feature is an ovoid or triangular hyperechoic mass located between the abdominal wall and the bowel, frequently in the right upper quadrant (**Figure 7**) [3]. In some cases, avascular hypoechoic tubular structure can be seen corresponds to a twisted vein. Although, some centers recommend conservative treatment, others prefer surgery to remove the necrotic tissue [24].

14. Inguinal hernia

In the setting of a groin mass or swelling, possible diagnoses are hernia, fluid collection, enlarged lymph nodes, and cryptorchidism, and for those US can be performed to differentiate. The most common type of inguinal hernia in children is the indirect inguinal hernia in which hernia sac protrude into the inguinal canal [41]. Inguinal hernia is more common in preterm neonates and more frequently occurs on the right side because the right processus vaginalis closes later than the left. One-third of all infants with hernias become symptomatic before 6 months after birth, and males are affected more than females with a ratio of 6:1 [58]. Hernia sac frequently includes fluid in the processus vaginalis with or without bowel loops and other abdominal structures such as omentum, testes, ovaries, bladder and fallopian tubes. If hernia sac contains intestine and other abdominal structures; possibility of spontaneous regression reduces and incarceration risk increases. Hence, early diagnosis and surgery is very important in order to prevent complications and possible damage to the ipsilateral testis [6, 58].

The diagnostic accuracy of US to detect inguinal hernia is 97% in surgically confirmed cases with the sensitivity of 92.7% and the specificity of 92.7% [6]. Internal inguinal canal diameter > 4 mm is 95% diagnostic for indirect inguinal hernia. Real-time imaging on US is the biggest advantage among other modalities, with the patient performing a Valsalva maneuver (or provoke to cry in infants or babies) in both supine and upright views that enlarge the hernia sac and protrude through the inguinal canal with increased intraabdominal pressure. US can also be able to reveal peristalsis of herniated bowel segment with dynamic scan. Large inguinal hernias may lead to testicular ischemia by compressing the gonadal vessels within the inguinal canal [59]. Therefore, ipsilateral testis should be evaluated with US and color Doppler to assess intratesticular blood flow in the setting of inguinal hernia. While, evaluating a patient with an inguinal hernia, US should be performed to both inguinal canals because a clinically occult contralateral hernia can be found in 88% of cases [58].

Incarceration is a remarkable complication of indirect inguinal hernia and occurs with a frequency of 31% in children [58]. The most common incarcerated contents of hernia sac are the bowel, ovaries, and fallopian tubes. An incarcerated inguinal hernia may gradually progress to a strangulation, in which vascular supply is compromised and the necrosis of incarcerated contents occur. On US, incarcerated bowel shows circumferential thickening of the wall, aperistalsis, fluid level in the herniated loop, free fluid in the hernia sac and intraabdominal bowel dilatation (**Figure 8**). Incarcerated or strangulated hernias may not demonstrate clear continuity with abdominal bowel loops. Color Doppler may demonstrate absent vascularity in the hernia sac as a late finding of strangulation [41]. The presence of peristaltic activity in the herniated bowel loop is strong evidence against strangulation.

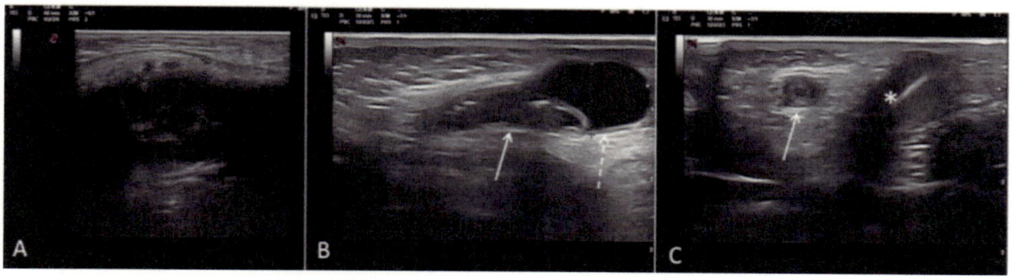

Figure 8.
Ultrasound of an indirect inguinal hernia of an 8-week-old baby (A,B,C). Along with bowel, blind ending appendix (arrow) is herniated into the inguinal canal, called as Amyand hernia. (B) There is some fluid (dashed arrow) within the hernia sac and (C) transverse section of distal appendix is seen at the same level with penile shaft (asterisk).

15. Foreign bodies and gastric bezoar

Coins are the most common foreign material ingested, and most of them are not able to reach intraabdominal GI tract [41]. Two-third of those is located at the level of cricopharyngeus muscle that requires urgent endoscopic removal. In the radiologic evaluation of the ingested foreign body, plain radiographs are frequently the modality of choice. Nevertheless, all foreign bodies are not visible on plain films, depending on composition of the material and location within the body. US may provide additional information about the foreign bodies trapped in the intraabdominal GI tract [60]. However, diagnostic performance of US to detect intraabdominal foreign body is not known to date. Most of the foreign bodies in bowel appear as fixed, hyperechoic structure that often demonstrate posterior acoustic shadowing with a cleaner shadow than bowel gas [6]. Linear, high frequency transducers should be used with graded compression to evaluate intraluminal contents. Administration of 200–300 mL of oral water before the examination may facilitate the detection of foreign bodies within the stomach [41].

A bezoar consists of ingested foreign objects that cluster within the GI tract. The most common types are trichobezoars (composed of hair) and phytobezoars (composed of greengrocer fibers) and they usually accumulate in the stomach [39]. Sometimes enlarged bezoars reach to the small bowel and cause obstruction. Prior history of gastric surgery is an important predisposing factor to develop bezoar due to delayed gastric emptying [41]. On US, regardless of the originated fiber, bezoar is shown as an intraluminal mass with hyperechoic arc-like (curved or "inverted U" shape) anterior surface and prominent acoustic shadowing (**Figure 9**). Color Doppler

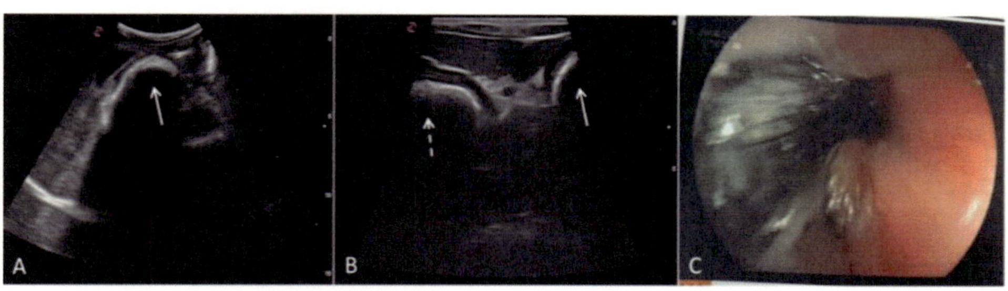

Figure 9.
A 12-year-old girl with a history of compulsive trichophagia disorder. Upper abdomen sonography with convex-array transducer (A) and linear-array transducer (B), demonstrates curvilinear echogenicities beneath the anterior wall of the stomach (arrow) and duodenum (dashed arrow) with clear, marked black posterior shadow. On endoscopy (C), trichobezoar was removed from her stomach and proximal duodenum.

can be used as a supportive modality which demonstrates 'twinkling artifact' behind the hyperechoic surface [39]. Bowel obstruction and proximal dilatation may be revealed as associated features.

16. Conclusion

While evaluating the etiology of acute abdominal pain in pediatric patients, US should be the initial imaging modality, as US is sufficient to diagnose several diseases that cause abdominal pain, far beyond only appendicitis and intussusception. Even if the underlying cause has not been identified, US will show indirect signs that indicate the need for a surgical exploration or provide supplemental information for CT and MRI. Therefore, it is crucial to be aware of the full potential of targeted bowel US with proper selection of the transducers, optimal positioning and the application of graded compression technique. Good quality examination requires experience, training, time and attention to perform a detailed evaluation of as many bowel loops as possible, minding their morphological features and their functional characteristics. Radiologists should be familiar with the sonographic appearance of both the normal and abnormal GI tract in order to provide the optimal treatment options for pediatric patients with acute abdominal diseases.

Acknowledgements

I thank Dr. Fatma Demirbas (Diyarbakır Children's Hospital) for providing endoscopic image of the trichobezoar case.

Author details

Ercan Ayaz
Department of Radiology, Diyarbakır Children's Hospital, Diyarbakır, Turkey

*Address all correspondence to: ercan.ayaz1@gmail.com

References

[1] Esposito F, Di Serafino M, Mercogliano C, Ferrara D, Vezzali N, Di Nardo G, et al. The pediatric gastrointestinal tract: ultrasound findings in acute diseases. Journal of Ultrasound 2019;22:409-422. DOI: 10.1007/s40477-018-00355-0

[2] Nylund K, Maconi G, Hollerweger A, Ripolles T, Pallotta N, Higginson A, et al. EFSUMB Recommendations and Guidelines for Gastrointestinal Ultrasound Part 1: Examination Techniques and Normal Findings (Long version). Ultraschall in Med 2017;38:e1-15. DOI: 10.1055/s-0042-115853.

[3] Hwang JY. Emergency ultrasonography of the gastrointestinal tract of children. Ultrasonography 2017;36:204-221. DOI: 10.1055/s-0042-115853

[4] Riccabona M, Lobo ML, Augdal TA, Avni F, Blickman J, Bruno C, et al. European Society of Paediatric Radiology Abdominal Imaging Task Force recommendations in paediatric uroradiology, part X: how to perform paediatric gastrointestinal ultrasonography, use gadolinium as a contrast agent in children, follow up paediatric testicular microlithiasis, and an update on paediatric contrast-enhanced ultrasound. Pediatric Radiology.2018;48:1528-1536. DOI: 10.1007/s00247-018-4147-3

[5] Lobo ML, Roque M. Gastrointestinal ultrasound in neonates, infants and children. Eur J Radiol. 2014;83: 1592-1600. DOI: 10.1016/j.ejrad.2014.04.016.

[6] Anupindi SA, Halverson M, Khwaja A, Jeckovic M, Wang X, Bellah RD. Common and Uncommon Applications of Bowel Ultrasound With Pathologic Correlation in Children. AJR 2014; 202:946-959. DOI: 10.2214/AJR.13.11661.

[7] Havre R, Gilja OH. Elastography and strain rate imaging of the gastrointestinal tract. Eur J Radiol 2014;83:438-441. DOI: 10.1016/j.ejrad.2013.05.018.

[8] Giannetti A, Biscontri M, Matergi M. Feasibility of real-time strain elastography in colonic diseases. J Ultrasound 2014; 17: 321-330. DOI: 10.1007/s40477-014-0124-3

[9] Baumgart DC, Muller HP, Grittner U, Metzke D, Fischer A, Guckelberger O, et al. US-based Real-time Elastography for the Detection of Fibrotic Gut Tissue in Patients with Stricturing Crohn Disease. Radiology 2015; 275: 889-899. DOI: 10.1148/radiol.14141929

[10] Fraquelli M, Branchi F, Cribiu FM, Orlando S, Casazza G, Magarotto A, et al. The Role of Ultrasound Elasticity Imaging in Predicting Ileal Fibrosis in Crohn's Disease Patients. Inflamm Bowel Dis 2015; 21: 2605-2612. DOI: 10.1097/MIB.0000000000000536.

[11] Frohlich E, Muller R, Cui XW, Schreiber-Dietrich D, Dietrich CF. Dynamic contrast-enhanced ultrasound for quantification of tissue perfusion. J Ultrasound Med 2015; 34: 179-196. DOI: 10.7863/ultra.34.2.179.

[12] Incesu L, Yazicioglu AK, Selcuk MB, Ozen N. Contrast-enhanced power Doppler US in the diagnosis of acute appendicitis. Eur J Radiol 2004; 50: 201-209. DOI: 10.1016/S0720-048X(03)00102-5.

[13] Ripolles T, Martinez-Perez MJ, Paredes JM, García-Martínez E, Jiménez-Restrepo DH. Contrast-enhanced ultrasound in the differentiation between phlegmon and abscess in Crohn's disease and other abdominal conditions. Eur J Radiol 2013; 82: e525-e531. DOI: 10.1016/j.ejrad.2013.05.043.

[14] Puylaert JB. Acute appendicitis: US evaluation using graded compression. Radiology 1986; 158: 355-360. DOI: 10.1148/radiology.158.2.2934762.

[15] Lameris W, van RA, Bipat S, Bossuyt PM, Boermeester MA, Stoker J. Graded compression ultrasonography and computed tomography in acute colonic diverticulitis: meta-analysis of test accuracy. Eur Radiol 2008; 18: 2498-2511. DOI: 10.1007/s00330-008-1018-6.

[16] Parra DA, Navarro OM. Sonographic diagnosis of intestinal polyps in children. Pediatr Radiol 2008; 38: 680-684. DOI: 10.1007/s00247-008-0812-2

[17] Pallotta N, Baccini F, Corazziari E. Ultrasonography of the small bowel after oral administration of anechoic contrast solution. Lancet 1999; 353: 985-986. DOI: 10.1016/S0140-6736(98)05504-4.

[18] Blumfield E, Levin TL, Kurian J, Lee EY, Liszewski MC. Imaging Findings in Multisystem Inflammatory Syndrome in Children (MIS-C) Associated With Coronavirus Disease (COVID-19). AJR 2021; 216:507-518. DOI: 10.2214/AJR.20.24032.

[19] Chiorean L, Schreiber-Dietrich D, Braden B, Cui X, Dietrich CF. Transabdominal ultrasound for standardized measurement of bowel wall thickness in normal children and those with Crohn's disease. Med Ultrason 2014; 16: 319-324. DOI: 10.11152/mu.201.3.2066.164.dsd2.

[20] Nylund K, Hausken T, Ødegaard S, Eide GE, Gilja OH. Gastrointestinal wall thickness measured with transabdominal ultrasonography and its relationship to demographic factors in healthy subjects. Ultraschall in Med. 2012; 33: E225–E232. DOI: 10.1055/s-0031-1299329.

[21] Ferri E, Bonvicini U, Pisani M. Ultrasonography of normal vermiform appendix. Chir Ital. 2001; 53: 231-238.

[22] di Giacomo V, Trinci M, van der Byl G, Catania VD, Calisti A, Miele V. Ultrasound in newborns and children suffering from non-traumatic acute abdominal pain: imaging with clinical and surgical correlation. J Ultrasound. 2014;18:385-393. DOI: 10.1007/s40477-014-0087-4

[23] Sargar KM, Siegel MJ. Sonography of acute appendicitis and its mimics in children. Indian J Radiol Imaging. 2014;24:163-170. DOI: 10.4103/0971-3026.134404.

[24] Munden MM, Hill JG. Ultrasound of the acute abdomen in children. Ultrasound Clin. 2010;5:113-135. DOI: 10.1016/j.cult.2009.11.016

[25] Dirks K, Calabrese E, Dietrich CF, Gilja OH, Hausken T, Higginson A, et al. EFSUMB Position Paper: Recommendations for Gastrointestinal Ultrasound (GIUS) in Acute Appendicitis and Diverticulitis. Ultraschall in Med. 2019;40:163-175. DOI: 10.1055/a-0824-6952.

[26] Quigley AJ, Stafrace S. Ultrasound assessment of acute appendicitis in paediatric patients: methodology and pictorial overview of findings seen. Insights Imaging. 2013;4:741-751. DOI: 10.1007/s13244-013-0275-3

[27] Chang ST, Jeffrey RB, Olcott EW. Three-step sequential positioning algorithm during sonographic evaluation for appendicitis increases appendiceal visualization rate and reduces CT use. Am J Roentgenol. 2014;203:1006-1012. DOI: 10.2214/Am J Roentgenol.13.12334

[28] Birnbaum BA, Jeffrey RB Jr. CT and sonographic evaluation of acute right lower quadrant abdominal pain. Am J

Roentgenol. 1998;170:361-371. DOI: 10.2214/ajr.170.2.9456947

[29] Chicaiza HP, Malia L, Mulvey CH, Smith SR. Revisiting the Appendiceal Diameter via Ultrasound for the Diagnosis of Acute Appendicitis. Pediatric emergency care 2017. DOI: 10.1097/pec.0000000000001278

[30] Xu Y, Jeffrey RB, Chang ST, DiMaio MA, Olcott EW. Sonographic Differentiation of Complicated From Uncomplicated Appendicitis: Implications for Antibiotics- First Therapy. J Ultrasound Med 2017; 36: 269-277. DOI: 10.7863/ultra.16.03109

[31] Rodriguez DP, Vargas S, Callahan MJ, Zurakowski D, Taylor GA. Appendicitis in young children: imaging experience and clinical outcomes. AJR Am J Roentgenol 2006;186:1158-1164. DOI: 10.2214/AJR.05.0055.

[32] Hollerweger A. Acute appendicitis: sonographic evaluation. Ultraschall in Med. 2006; 27: 412– 426. DOI: 10.1055/s-2006-927118-2

[33] Partain KN, Patel A, Travers C, McCracken CE, Loewen J, Braithwaite K, et al. Secondary signs may improve the diagnostic accuracy of equivocal ultrasounds for suspected appendicitis in children. Journal of pediatric surgery 2016; 51: 1655-1660. DOI: 10.1016/j.jpedsurg.2016.03.005

[34] Bhangu A, Søreide K, Di Saverio S, Assarsson JH, Drake FT. Acute appendicitis: modern understanding of pathogenesis, diagnosis, and management. The Lancet. 2015;386:1278-1287. DOI: 10.1016/s0140-6736(15)00275-5

[35] Dibble EH, Swenson DW, Cartagena C, Baird GL, Herliczek TW. Effectiveness of a Staged US and Unenhanced MR Imaging Algorithm in the Diagnosis of Pediatric Appendicitis. Radiology. 2017. DOI: 10.1148/radiol.2017162755

[36] Benabbas R, Hanna M, Shah J, Sinert R. Diagnostic Accuracy of History, Physical Examination, Laboratory Tests, and Point-of-care Ultrasound for Pediatric Acute Appendicitis in the Emergency Department: A Systematic Review and Meta-analysis. Academic emergency medicine: official journal of the Society for Academic Emergency Medicine. 2017;24:523-551. DOI:10.1111/acem.13181

[37] Atema JJ, Gans SL, Van Randen A, Laméris W, van Es HW, van Heesewijk JP, et al. Comparison of Imaging Strategies with Conditional versus Immediate Contrast-Enhanced Computed Tomography in Patients with Clinical Suspicion of Acute Appendicitis. Eur Radiol. 2015; 25: 2445-2452. DOI: 10.1007/s00330-015-3648-9

[38] Gorter RR, Eker HH, Gorter-Stam MA, Abis GS, Acharya A, Ankersmit M, et al. Diagnosis and management of acute appendicitis. EAES consensus development conference 2015. Surg Endosc. 2016;30:4668-4690. DOI:10.1007/s00464-016-5245-7

[39] Arys B, Mandelstam S, Rao P, Kernick S, Kumbla S. Sonography of the Pediatric Gastrointestinal System. Ultrasound Quarterly. 2014;30:101-117. DOI: 10.1097/RUQ.0b013e3182a38dcc.

[40] Niedzielski J, Kobielski A, Sokal J, Krakos M. Accuracy of sonographic criteria in the decision for surgical treatment in infantile hypertrophic pyloric stenosis. Arch Med Sci. 2011;7:508-511. DOI: 10.5114/aoms.2011.23419

[41] Gale HI, Gee MS, Westra SJ, Nimkin K. Abdominal ultrasonography

of the pediatric gastrointestinal tract. World J Radiol. 2016;8:656-667. DOI: 10.4329/wjr.v8.i7.656.

[42] Menke J, Kahl F. Sonography-guided hydrostatic reduction of ileocolic intussusception in children: analysis of failure and success in consecutive patients presenting timely to the hospital. Eur J Pediatr. 2015;174:307-316. DOI: 10.1007/s0043 1-014-2394-3

[43] Navarro O, Dugougeat F, Kornecki A, Shuckett B, Alton DJ, Daneman A. The impact of imaging in the management of intussusception owing to pathologic lead points in children: a review of 43 cases. Pediatr Radiol. 2000;30:594-603. DOI: 10.1007/s002470000261

[44] Shalaby MS, Kuti K, Walker G. Intestinal malrotation and volvulus in infants and children. BMJ. 2013;26:347. DOI: 10.1136/bmj.f6949

[45] Karmazyn B. Duodenum between the aorta and the SMA does not exclude malrotation. Pediatr Radiol. 2013;43:121-122. DOI: 10.1007/s00247-012-2537-5.

[46] Epelman M, Daneman A, Navarro OM, Morag I, Moore AM, Kim JH, et al. Necrotizing enterocolitis: review of state-of-the-art imaging findings with pathologic correlation. Radiographics. 2007;27:285-305. DOI: 10.1148/rg.272055098

[47] Faingold R, Daneman A, Tomlinson G, Babyn PS, Manson DE, Mohanta A, et al. Necrotizing enterocolitis: assessment of bowel viability with color Doppler US. Radiology. 2005; 235:587-594. DOI: 10.1148/radiol.2352031718

[48] Kim WY, Kim WS, Kim IO, Kwon TH, Chang W, Lee EK. Sonographic evaluation of neonates with early-stage necrotizing enterocolitis. Pediatr Radiol. 2005;35:1056-1061. DOI: 10.1007/s00247-005-1533-4.

[49] Silva CT, Daneman A, Navarro O, Moineddin R, Levine D, Moore AM. A prospective comparison of intestinal sonography and abdominal radiographs in a neonatal intensive care unit. Pediatr Radiol. 2013;43:1453-1463. DOI: 10.1007/s00247-013-2777-z

[50] Spalinger J, Patriquin H, Miron MC, Marx G, Herzog D, Dubois J, et al. Doppler US in patients with Crohn disease: vessel density in the diseased bowel reflects disease activity. Radiology 2000; 217:787-791. DOI: 10.1148/radiology.217.3.r00dc19787

[51] Alison M, Kheniche A, Azoulay R, Roche S, Sebag G, Belarbi N. Ultrasonography of Crohn disease in children. Pediatr Radiol 2007; 37:1071-1082. DOI: 10.1007/s00247-007-0559-1

[52] Trapani S, Micheli A, Grisolia F, Resti M, Chiappini E, Falcini F, et al. Henoch Schonlein purpura in childhood: epidemiological and clinical analysis of 150 cases over a 5-year period and review of literature. Semin Arthritis Rheum 2005;35:143-153. DOI: 10.1016/j.semarthrit.2005.08.007

[53] Hryhorczuk AL, Lee EY. Imaging evaluation of bowel obstruction in children: updates in imaging techniques and review of imaging findings. Semin Roentgenol. 2012;47:159-170. DOI: 10.1053/j.ro.2011.11.007

[54] Kılıç Ö, Somer A, Hançerli Törün S, Keser Emiroğlu M, Salman N, Salman T, et al. Assessment of 35 children with abdominal tuberculosis. Turk J Gastroenterol 2015; 26: 128-132. DOI: 10.5152/tjg.2015.6123

[55] Dietrich CF, Hermann S, Klein S, Braden B. Sonographic signs of neutropenic enterocolitis. World J Gastroenterol. 2006;12:1397-1402. DOI: 10.3748/wjg.v12.i9.1397

[56] Simanovsky N, Hiller N. Importance of sonographic detection of enlarged abdominal lymph nodes in children. J Ultrasound Med 2007;26:581-584. DOI: 10.7863/jum.2007.26.5.581

[57] Singh AK, Gervais DA, Hahn PF, Sagar P, Mueller PR, Novelline RA. Acute epiploic appendagitis and its mimics. Radiographics. 2005;25:1521-1534. DOI: 10.1148/rg.256055030

[58] Meena D, Jhuria R, Saxena S, Saini U. Inguinoscrotal hernia in infants: Three case reports in ultrasound diagnosis. Indian J Radiol Imaging. 2017;27:78-81. DOI: 10.4103/0971-3026.202951

[59] Orth RC, Towbin AJ. Acute testicular ischemia caused by incarcerated inguinal hernia. Pediatr Radiol 2012;42:196-200. DOI: 10.1007/s00247-011-2210-4

[60] Halverson M, Servaes S. Foreign bodies: radiopaque compared to what? Pediatr Radiol 2013; 43:1103-1107. DOI: 10.1007/s00247-013-2660-y.

Chapter 3

Ultrasound Modality in the Evaluation and Management of Gallbladder Polyps

Haithem Zaafouri, Meryam Mesbahi, Nizar Khedhiri, Wassim Riahi, Mouna Cherif, Dhafer Haddad and Anis Ben Maamer

Abstract

Gallbladder polyps (GBP) are defined as developed masses inside the wall of the gallbladder; most of them (90%) are nontumor lesions. Abdominal ultrasound is the main and the first line radiological modality for their diagnosis and their risk lamination. We conducted a 12 year retrospective study between 2009 and 2020, which included patients who had preoperative transabdominal ultrasonography showing gallbladder polyps and had undergone cholecystectomy, and for whom postoperative pathology results were available, as well as patients who had at least one polyp discovered on the histopathological exam and who were not determined preoperatively. A total of 70 patients were identified. Preoperative diagnosis of vesicular polyp by ultrasound was carried in 82.9% of patients. The number of ultrasounds performed per person was 1.2 ± 0.47. The polyps' size in mm was on average 6.14 ± 2.6 with extremes between 3 and 13 mm. On anatomopathological examination, a polyp was objectified in 33.3% of cases. In our series, abdominal ultrasound had a low sensitivity at 36.4%. We aim to provide the accuracy of abdominal ultrasound for the diagnosis of GBP, as a low-cost modality, and to evaluate the concordance of preoperative ultrasound imaging with postoperative pathology.

Keywords: gallbladder polyps, abdominal ultrasound, sensitivity, cholecystectomy, management

1. Introduction

Gallbladder polyps (GBP) are defined as developed masses inside the wall of the gallbladder; most of them (90%) are nontumor lesions [1]. They have been firstly classified in 1976 as benign tumors, pseudotumors, and malignant tumors [2].

Abdominal ultrasound is the main and the first line radiological modality for their diagnosis and their risk lamination [3]. It has been proven in the literature, the superiority of ultrasound by comparing it to other imaging techniques such as CT scan [4].

Ultrasound diagnosis of GBP is founded on two criteria—the lack of posterior acoustic shadow and immobility when changing the patient's position [1, 5].

Transabdominal ultrasound represents also an essential modality for the follow-up of GBP [6].

Nowadays, plenty of radiological modalities, such as transabdominal ultrasonography, endoscopic ultrasonography, magnetic resonance imaging (MRI), CT scan, or PET-CT have been employed for the diagnosis of GBP [7].

GBP are potentially malignant lesions so that it is mandatory to be precise whether the polyp is a high or low risk of malignancy and to lead undoubtedly to their perfect management [8].

We aim to provide the accuracy of abdominal ultrasound for the diagnosis of GBP, as a low-cost modality, and to evaluate the concordance of preoperative ultrasound imaging with postoperative pathology.

2. Methods

We conducted a 12 year retrospective study between 2009 and 2020, which included patients who had preoperative transabdominal ultrasonography showing gallbladder polyps and had undergone cholecystectomy, and for whom postoperative pathology results were available, as well as patients who had at least one polyp discovered on the histopathological exam and who were not determined preoperatively.

Epidemiological, clinical, morphological, and ultrasound data were then collected, as well as data from anatomy pathology interventions and reports.

3. Results

A total of 70 patients were identified. The sex ratio (male:female) was 0.34. The average age was 53.4 years with extremes ranging from 28 to 78 years. A total of 35 patients had a medical history, such as high blood pressure (25.7%), dyslipidemia (11.4%), and diabetes (8.6%). A total of 45 patients had a surgical history. The ASA score was 1 in 62.9%, 2 in 34.3%, and 3 in 2.9%.

Abdominal ultrasound was performed in all patients.

Preoperative diagnosis of vesicular polyp by ultrasound was carried in 82.9% of patients. Either due to symptoms in 68.6% of cases—right hypochondrium pain (48.4%), liver colic (35.5%), vomiting (9.7%) or fortuitous discovery in 8.6% of cases during an abdominal ultrasound for other pathology, or systematically in 5.7% of cases (four cases) as part of the preoperative assessment of an umbilical hernia.

In 17.1% of cases, the polyp was discovered perioperatively.

The number of ultrasounds performed per person was 1.2 ± 0.47.

Characteristics	
Age (years)	53.4
Symptoms, (%)	68.8%
Diabetes mellitus	8.6%
Size of gallbladder polyp (mm)	6.14 ± 2.6
No. of polyps per patient	1.59 ± 0.79
Coexistin ggallstones	4

Table 1.
Demographic and clinical characteristics of the study population.

The number of gallbladder polyps per patient was 1.59 ± 0.79.

The polyps' size in mm was on average 6.14 ± 2.6 with extremes between 3 and 13 mm. Gallbladder polyp and gallbladder stones were found in four patients (**Table 1**).

Other additional tests were performed: abdominal CT scan in 17.1% of cases, MRI in 5.7% of cases, upper endoscopy in 14.3% of cases, especially before gastric pain.

The surgical indication was retained especially when there were symptomatic polyps whatever the size, which was in 67.6% of cases.

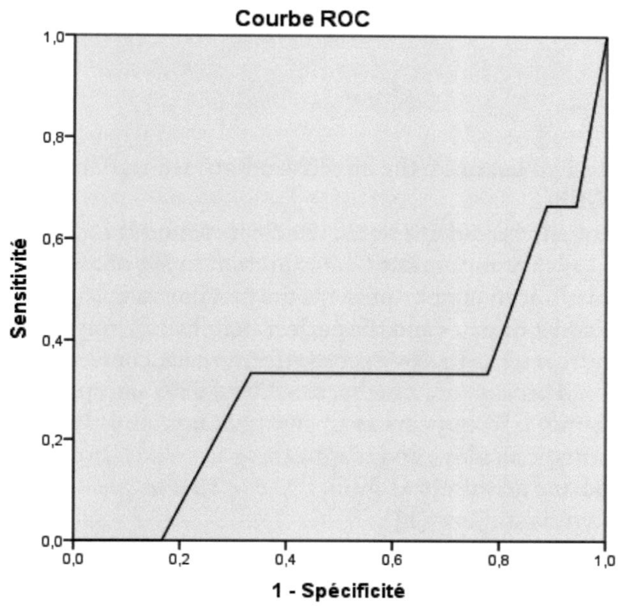

Figure 1.
Correlation between the size of the polyp on the abdominal ultrasound and the presence of polyp on the piece of cholecystectomy.

Positive if >=	Sensibility	Specificity
2.00	1000	1000
3.35	667	944
3.85	667	889
4.25	333	778
4.75	333	722
5.25	333	611
5.75	333	556
7.00	333	333
8.25	000	167
9.75	000	111
12.00	000	056
14.00	000	000

Table 2.
Sensibility and specificity of the abdominal ultrasound in function of the size of the polyp.

Cholecystectomy was performed by laparoscopy in 82.9% of cases.

On anatomopathological examination, a polyp was objectified in 33.3% of cases. The average size was 8.83 ± 10.8 mm. Dysplasia was found in 72.7% of all polyps.

In 22.7% of cases, cholesterolosis was noted.

In our series, abdominal ultrasound had a low sensitivity at 36.4%.

Using the ROC curve (**Figure 1**) to study the correlation between the size of the polyp on the abdominal ultrasound and the presence of polyp on the piece of cholecystectomy, we found that the area under the curve was 0.315, which corresponds to a low discriminating power.

The study of the coordinates of the curve showed that a size of 7 mm would have the best specificity and sensitivity (**Table 2**).

4. Discussion

This cohort study is based on the effectiveness of transabdominal ultrasound on the detection of GBP.

GBP is the frequent vesicular lesions, which are found frequently on abdominal ultrasonography [8]. Asymptomatic GBP is present in 5% of adults [9].

The abdominal ultrasonography presents the first line radiological means for the diagnosis of gallbladder diseases and the perfect examination for diagnosing polyps [4, 8]. Considering that it has the lower cost-effectiveness, convenient accessibility, the lack of radiation, and because of its higher sensitivity 93% and specificity 95.3% [8–10].

On the ultrasound, GBP appears as an elevated, immobile lesion of the wall, it has a posterior acoustic shadow, and it appears as a sessile lesion [11, 12].

Despite the routine use of ultrasound, it seems that its positive predictive value in diagnosing polyps is still low [13].

It can present some limitations because it is operator-dependent [14], and it can provide errors in the determination of polyps, their numbers, and their size [8].

As an example, a gallstone can be easily mistaken for a polyp on ultrasonography [15], as it can be only identified on ultrasound if it measures over 5 mm [15].

Many hypotheses have been studied to explain the poor sensitivity of ultrasound in determining true polyps, Kratzer proposed in this case, that the initial diagnosis of a polyp might be incorrect [7]. As seen in the Cochrane review that the cause of false diagnoses by ultrasound was generally a result of misinterpretation of gallstones as polyps [10].

However, Ostapenko [13] has concluded that seven patients of 34 with GBP did not have a detectable polyp, supporting the argument that the initial diagnosis was a false positive.

In our series, ultrasound had a sensitivity of 36.4%. Several factors could explain this result. Since ultrasound is a dependent operator examination, gall bladder stones, especially those of small size, could be taken on account of a polyp. The polyp's migration to the bile ducts could be another explanation and would probably be the cause of the hepatic colic. The absence of polyp on the histological examination could also be explained by the manipulation of the gallbladder during cholecystectomy.

In case of diagnostic difficulties, and mainly when malignancy is suspected, other complementary investigations can be more helpful [14, 16, 17] presenting by:

Contrast-enhanced sonography: which is an ultrasound enhanced by the injection of a medium non-irradiating ultrasonic contrast (microbubbles), is more specific in the study of vascularity, showing hyper-echoic contrast during the arterial phase and iso-echoic images during the venous phase. So, it is more useful to identify gallbladder polyps of multiple stones and from other polypoid lesions [9, 14].

Magnetic resonance imaging (MRI): It is a particular modality used in the differentiation between gallbladder polyps from other polypoid lesions, especially adenomyomatosis [14].

Positron emission tomography (PET): It is used to evaluate the malignancy diagnosis in polyps rising more than 10 mm by hypermetabolism [14].

Endoscopic ultrasound (EUS): It is determined to be better than ultrasound, it is the best modality in diagnosing gallbladder polyps [15], especially when there is suspicion of regional lymph nodes, providing the staging of polypoid lesions [14, 15].

Conventional ultrasound is sufficient to investigate GBP compared to other modalities, however, it has been proven in some studies that endoscopic ultrasound is more specific and exact, especially in the differentiation between true and pseudopolyps [11].

Guo [8] confirmed the accuracy of ultrasound for polyps diagnosis which was 78.8% in their work, and its accuracy for differentiation between benign and malignant polyps, which was confirmed in the Cochrane review [10]. Our results are in line with these cohort studies.

On ultrasonography, the polyp echogenicity is used to distinguish between true, pseudopolyps, and gallstones [18].

Its main role is to identify prematurely the progression of polyps to malignant carcinomas [13]. Polyps size is considered the main indicator of potential malignancy [16].

According to the guidelines, an arbitrary cut-off of 10 mm is confirmed to indicate cholecystectomy, which is justified by the increased incidence of gallbladder carcinoma in the polyps rising sharply from 10 mm and upwards [11, 16, 18, 19].

Polyps can cause symptoms and the relationship between symptoms and risk of malignancy is still controversial according to the literature, so cholecystectomy is wisely indicated when GBP are symptomatic [11].

Many factors that influence the therapeutic strategy of GBP were studied, including mainly the polyp size on radiological findings [18].

Referring to the literature (recent guidelines by the ESGAR group), the main factors that determine malignancy included primarily—the size greater than 10 mm, the sessile morphology, the presence of symptoms, the age 50 years and older, the Indian ethnicity, and the associated primary sclerosing cholangitis (**Figure 2**) [14, 18, 20].

Several retrospective studies showed controversial results about factors influencing malignancy and indicating cholecystectomy, which are—concomitant gallstones, elevated CA 19-9 marker, rapid polyp growth, and the number of polyps [14, 18, 20].

Gallbladder polyps are generally diagnosed and monitored by ultrasonography which is debated in the literature, discussing its accuracy [16]. Some studies confirmed its failure for the diagnosis, seen the absence of polyps at numerous histological examinations [16].

Several series have studied the correlation between ultrasound findings and histopathology results, concluded significant conjunction for the size determination between both modalities [15].

Elmasry [16] showed a significant number of gallbladder polyps that were not seen at histological examination postcholecystectomy, with an incidence of 16.4% of all histological results. This can be explained that polyps may be destroyed by the mechanical action of the gallbladder wall [7].

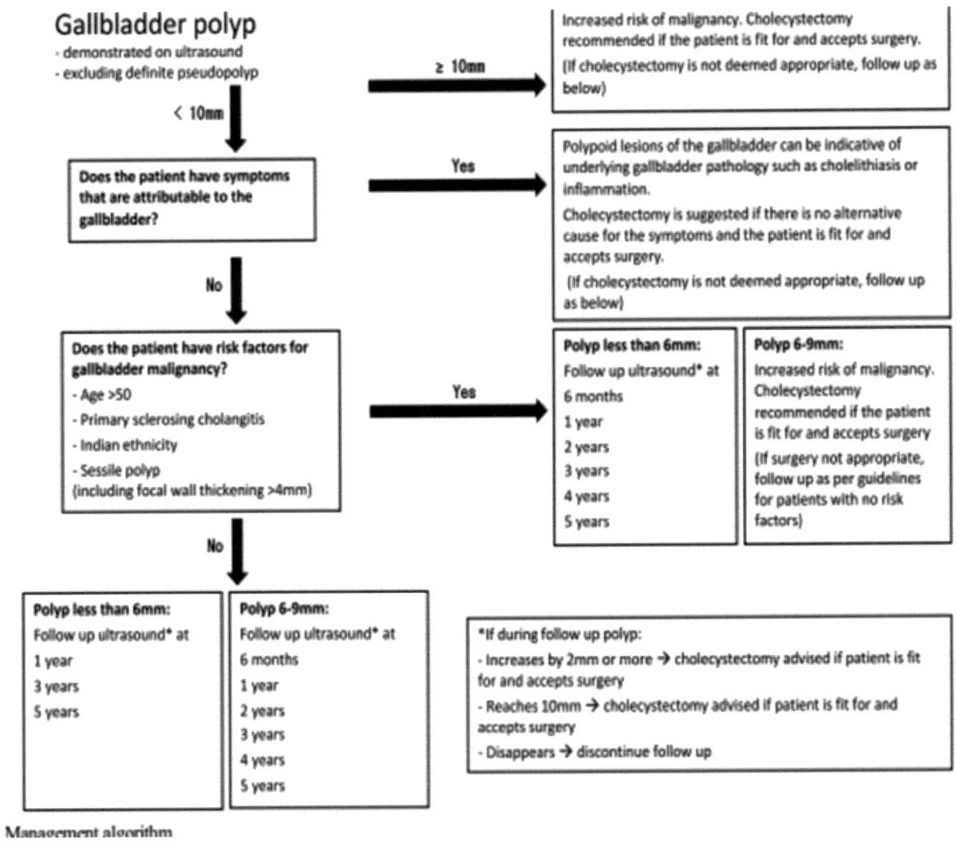

Figure 2.
Management algorithm for gallbladder polyps [11].

Nonresected GBP which are smaller than 10 mm are recommended to be followed up regularly with serial ultrasound imagery [15], every 6 months–1 year for those under 5 mm, every 3–6 months for those with a dimension of 5–10 mm [1].

Follow-up strategy of GBP is not yet based on any consensus on the size of polyps, neither on its frequency or duration. Recently, the guidelines of ESGAR states recommend that polyps of 6–9 mm should be supervised prudently than polyps of less than 6 mm [18]. So that the measurement of polyps size is mandatory during the follow up of GBP—it was found that 6.9% of polyps increased their size during the monitoring period [12].

It has been proven that there was no evidence data published to define the increasing size of the polyps during surveillance, which may be an indicator for cholecystectomy [2].

5. Conclusion

Preoperative diagnosis of GBP distinguishing malignant from benign lesions is challenging. Literature has highlighted the accuracy of ultrasound as the key modality for GBP detection.

It is used to be the gold standard, seeing it has relatively low-cost, low-risk, and widely available techniques. However, many studies discussed its ineffectiveness in polyp diagnosis, despite its major role in European guidelines. Leading to the essential role of other modalities such as magnetic resonance imaging, and endoscopic ultrasound. In the upcoming, studies should investigate more on the utility of these newer imaging techniques to enhance a new multimodal strategy to gallbladder polyp investigation.

Author details

Haithem Zaafouri*, Meryam Mesbahi, Nizar Khedhiri, Wassim Riahi, Mouna Cherif, Dhafer Haddad and Anis Ben Maamer
Department of General Surgery, Habib Thameur Hospital, Tunis, Tunisia

*Address all correspondence to: zaafouri.haithem@hotmail.fr

References

[1] Pirraci DA. Evaluation and Ultrasound Follow-up of Gallbladder Polyps. Webmed Central Radiology. 2013;**4**(6):WMC004297

[2] Morera-Ocón FJ, Ballestín-Vicente J, Calatayud-Blas AM, Cataldo de Tursi-Rispoli L, Bernal-Sprekelsen JC. Surgical indications in gallbladder polyps Cirugía Española. 2013;**91**(5): 324-330

[3] Choi TW. Risk stratification of gallbladder polyps larger than 10 mm using high-resolution ultrasonography and texture analysis. European Radiology. 2018;**28**(1):196-205

[4] Liu L-N, Xu H-X, Lu M-D, Xie X-Y, Wang W-P, Hu B, et al. Contrast-enhanced ultrasound in the diagnosis of gallbladder diseases: A multi-center experience. PLoS One. 2012;**7**(10):13

[5] Bae JS. Quantitative contrast-enhanced US helps differentiating neoplastic vs non-neoplastic gallbladder polyps. European Radiology. 2019; **29**(7):3772-3781

[6] Martin E, Gill R, Debru E. Diagnostic accuracy of transabdominal ultrasonography for gallbladder polyps: Systematic review. Canadian Journal of Surgery. 2018;**61**(3):200-207

[7] Kratzer W, Haenle MM, Voegtle A, Mason RA, Akinli AS, Hirschbuehl K, et al. Ultrasonographically detected gallbladder polyps: A reason for concern? A seven-year follow-up study. BMC Gastroenterology. 2008;**8**:41-49

[8] Guo J, Wu G, Zhou Z. Polypoid lesions of the gallbladder: report of 160 cases with special reference to diagnosis and treatment in China. International Journal of Clinical and Experimental Pathology. 2015;**8**(9):11569-11578

[9] Yuan Z. Is contrast-enhanced ultrasound superior to computed tomography for differential diagnosis of gallbladder polyps? A cross-sectional study. Frontiers in Oncology. 2021;**11**:12

[10] Sarah ZW, Mark PL, Marcello DM, Joost Ph D, Kurinchi SG, Cornelis Jhm van L. et al. Transabdominal ultrasound and endoscopic ultrasound for diagnosis of gallbladder polyps (review). Cochrane Database of Systematic Reviews. 2018;**8**(8):CD012233

[11] Wiles R. Management and follow-up of gallbladder polyps. European Radiology. 2017;**27**(9):3856-3866.

[12] Rafaelsen SR, Otto PO, Pedersen MRV. Long-term ultrasound follow-up in patients with small gallbladder polyps. Danish Medical Journal. 2020;**67**(10):1-7

[13] Ostapenko A, Liechty S, Kim M, Kleiner D. Accuracy of ultrasound in diagnosing gallbladder polyps at a community hospital. JSLS. 2020; **24**(4):1-5

[14] Valibouze C. The management of gallbladder polyps. Journal of Visceral Surgery 2020;**157**(5):410-417

[15] Andrén-Sandberg Å. Diagnosis and management of gallbladder polyps. North American Journal of Medicine and Science. 2012;**4**(5):10

[16] Elmasry MM, Mrcs M. The risk of malignancy in ultrasound detected gallbladder polyps: A systematic review. International Journal of Surgery. 2016;**33**:28-35

[17] Babu BI, Dennison AR, Garcea G. Management and diagnosis of gallbladder polyps: A systematic review. Langenbeck's Archives of Surgery. 2015;**400**(4):455-62

[18] McCain RS, Diamond A, Jones C, Coleman HG. Current practices and future prospects for the management of gallbladder polyps: A topical review. World Journal of Gastroenterology. 2018;**24**(26):2844-2852

[19] Jeong Y, Kim JH, Chae HD, Park SJ, Bae JS, Joo I, et al. Deep learning-based decision support system for the diagnosis of neoplastic gallbladder polyps on ultrasonography: Preliminary results. Scientific Reports 2020;**10**(1): 1-10

[20] Sun Y, Yang Z, Lan X, Tan H. Neoplastic polyps in gallbladder: A retrospective study to determine risk factors and treatment strategy for gallbladder polyps. Hepatobiliary Surgery and Nutrition. 2019;**8**(3):9

Chapter 4

Perspective Chapter: Recent Advances in Musculo-Skeletal Ultrasound

Felix Okechukwu Erondu

Abstract

Medical imaging specialists continue to explore better ways of demonstrating pathology and anatomy of the musculo-skeletal system. The continuous quest is fuelled by the desire to improve diagnostic yield, perform procedures more quickly and accurately, reduce risks to patient or operator, achieve better cost efficiency and utilize less complex methodologies. In many instances, musculoskeletal ultrasound acts as a screening, diagnostic tool but also guide and monitor therapeutic interventions. The paper outlines the use of ultrasound in the imaging of peripheral nerve disorders, traumatic and atraumatic joint disorders, Doppler techniques such as super micro vascular Imaging and sono-elastography. Refinements in probe technology and application of digital and novel proprietary software, have continued to improve the resolution of ultrasound images and with finer details on a scale not previously possible. With increasing experience and standardization of protocols, Musculoskeletal ultrasound will continue to play a great role in the diagnostic work-up and treatment of related disorders.

Keywords: medical imaging, musculoskeletal, ultrasound, nerve imaging

1. Introduction

Medical imaging specialists continue to explore better ways of demonstrating pathology and anatomy of the musculo-skeletal system. The continuous quest is fuelled by the desire to improve diagnostic yield, perform procedures more quickly and accurately, reduce risks to patient or operator, achieve better cost efficiency and utilize less complex methodologies. The use of ultrasound in diagnosis of musculoskeletal disorders follows the same pattern; becoming an important and effective tool for the diagnosis and follow-up management of various disorders affecting the joints and soft tissues [1, 2].

Ultrasound meets the basic criteria for accuracy, safety, affordability and efficiency. The ability to perform studies in real time and thus possible correlation of physico-clinical features of disease entities are even more pertinent reasons to choose ultrasound. Furthermore, it holds a great potential in providing guide to therapy, allowing effective follow-up to be performed. It has also provided learning opportunities for a variety of practitioners in multiple specialties such as radiology, primary care, orthopedic surgery, podiatry and physiotherapy [3].

For physical therapists in particular, ultrasound provides a unique opportunity to have a real-time assessment of musculoskeletal system to identify changes in function, isolate pain following an injury and provide guide to useful interventions that can improve outcome [3]. In many climes, it can be argued that MRI is the mainstay modality in the evaluation of musculo-skeletal disorders. Its high cost, unavailability especially in developing and resource limited countries and the degree of sophistication required for its operation, remain reasons to explore ultrasound. Even when an MRI is available, diagnostic Ultrasound findings continue to play a complementary role in the diagnostic work-up.

Thankfully, the capabilities of ultrasound appear to have been enhanced by the presence of improved probe technology, better data acquisition and digital image processing techniques. Ultrasound has great potential for the imaging of tendons, nerves, ligaments, muscle tissue and adjoining joints [3–5].

The chapter is dedicated to reviewing various innovations and techniques of Musculo-skeletal ultrasound and promises to be useful to a wide range of readers.

2. The use of high resolution ultra-high frequency transducers

The improved diagnostic yield from ultrasound studies continues to fuel its utilization in the work up of various disease processes. In Particular, high resolution ultrasound is a requirement for musculo-skeletal imaging. To ensure that these requirements are in place, continuous research and development efforts are geared towards rapid advancements in electronics, computing, and transducer technology. Combined with sophisticated signal processing techniques, ultrasound has acquired the degree of spatial and contrast resolution required for musculo-skeletal imaging. The use of high-frequency transducers in the range of 12–18 MHz has become the mainstay in MSK ultrasound. The improved resolution afforded by this, allows evaluation of subtle changes in nerves, tendons, and ligaments [1, 4, 6]. Improvements in the design of ultrasound transducers has resulted in the development of those with very high frequency in the range of 20–70 MHz. This may have spatial resolution in the range of 50–100 μm, which permit detailed anatomy of the extremities. The higher the frequency, the better the spatial resolution and the less the penetrative ability of the resulting sound waves. Fortunately, deep penetration is not a critical requirement for superficial structures, thus ultra-high-frequency transducers are ideal for evaluating superficial musculoskeletal structures. In principle, what we lack in penetration, we gain in detail and spatial resolution. This sort of detail is invaluable when imaging the nerve fascicles by ultrasound [6–8].

3. Tendon/ligament imaging

Tendons are uniquely positioned to connect muscle tissue to bones. This is due to the high collagen content as well as the arrangement of fibers. Generally, the collagen macro-molecules are grouped into fibrils; an arrangement which is both layered and complex in nature. This in turn are bundled into fibers and fascicles surrounded by vascularized connective tissue endotendon. Each tendon is surrounded by a tendon sheath, made of two layers of synovium. Each tendon is uniquely suited to its function, and explains why the orientation of the fibers change, depending on how much tension it's expected to bear. Sometimes, the collagen is majorly aligned along the long axis of the tendon, as seen in the patella. In other tendons, particularly those with origins from more than one muscle such as the Achilles tendon and quadriceps tendon, the fibers run as discrete bundles. Although, healthy tendon bundles exhibit good tensile strength, repetitive stress may result in trauma to the tendon and tendinopathy. This is common in athletes, where acute inflammatory response may result in Paratenonitis or tenosynovitis. In contrast, ligaments are important in connecting two bones, and contain more proteoglycan and water, as well as a relatively lower collagen content. Furthermore, the connective tissue structure of ligaments are less uniform and consists of poorly ordered, interlaced and weaving pattern. Injuries to a ligament may cause further restriction of joint movement and therefore is associated with joint derangement. In imaging the ligament, it must be appreciated that the tension of each ligament may be determined by the extent of movement at the adjacent joint. The lesions which result from ligamental injury therefore depends on the position of the joint at the time of injury. The imaging of tendons and ligaments represents one of the best applications of musculoskeletal Ultrasound. It is not only accurate, but the timely diagnosis allows early intervention using conservative measures thereby delaying or reducing the likelihood of surgery) [9].

It is also possible to guide minimally invasive interventional treatments, which improves outcome and reduce the potential for post-intervention complications. In addition to all other advantages of ultrasound, the imaging of tendons is attractive due to a relatively high lesion detection rate [10]. The introduction of high-frequency, high resolution transducers, use of Doppler techniques and increasing information in this area, have improved the ability of ultrasound to detect fine textural abnormalities of these structures as well as to identify a variety of pathological conditions [11]. Ultrasound In tendon imaging, can evaluate the presence of dislocations, degenerative changes and tendon tears, longitudinal splits, partial and complete rupture, inflammatory conditions and tendon tumors. It is also invaluable as a tool to monitor healing after surgery and to identify post-surgical complications.

4. Nerve imaging

Imaging of the nervous and peripheral structures remain a challenge with conventional modalities such as X-rays and Computed tomography. Ultrasound provides an alternative and effective technique for imaging tendons and nerves. Its attraction is due to the fact that it is painless, has no known side effects and can actually be done in real-time examination. Non pathologic nerves are seen as continuous bundles of neuronal fascicle, which are separated from surrounding connective tissue [11, 12]. Ultrasound of the Neuro muscular tissues continue to define the diagnostic and treatment pathways for peripheral neuropathy [12]. The use of Standard transducers, will ensure imaging of a small proportion of nerve fascicles. This is seen as series of multiple hypoechoic parallel linear areas separated by echogenic bands, representing the fascicle and epineurium respectively. The latter is the outermost layer of dense irregular connective tissue surrounding a peripheral nerve. It usually surrounds multiple nerve fascicles as well as blood vessels which supply the nerve. When diseased, there are identifiable changes in the structure of the nerve tissues including disruption of the connective tissue, loss of parallel/linear hypoechoic fascicular architecture and swelling/increase in diameter. Compression of the nerve fascicles may occur with presence of cysts, tumors or aneurysmal dilatation of support vessels [11, 12].

A very common application of this technique is the evaluation of the relationships of median nerve anatomy in carpal tunnel syndrome, which may explain the cause of nerve compression or impingement. Sonographic changes include increase in the cross-sectional area of the nerve just proximal to the site of compression, loss of hyperechoic intensities within nerve as well as a reduction in mobility of the structures which it supplies [13, 14]. Ultrasound information supports clinical and electrophysiological testing for detection of compressing lesions caused by nerve entrapment in a variety of osteo-fibrous tunnels of the limbs and extremities. It is also possible to evaluate Congenital anomalies, nerve tears, and neurogenic tumors. Generally speaking, ultrasound has many advantages which include dynamic assessment, non-invasiveness, absence of pain and low cost of service. It therefore qualifies as both a screening, diagnostic as well as monitoring tool [12]. MRI provides a wider field of view, with 3- dimensional images when evaluating nerve entrapment, and the use of intravenous contrast, can diagnose persistent median artery. It is however more expensive, complex and time consuming. It may also have less diagnostic yield in children and patients with claustrophobia [12–14].

5. Sono-Elastography

Sono elastography has become increasingly useful in the evaluation of musculoskeletal disorder injuries and provides a non-invasive method of obtaining both qualitative and quantitative information of mechanical and structural properties of tissues [15]. When a tissue is subjected to a force within a defined cross-sectional area, it can experience changes in its structure or deformation. The degree of deformation is a function of how stiff the tissue is. The Tissue stiffness is expressed using a physical property called Young's modulus, or modulus of elasticity. Theoretically, Young's modulus is defined as the ratio of stress (the force per cross-sectional area) for a certain material and the strain (i.e. deformation; in this case, tissue deformation). The study of the elastic properties of tissues using ultrasound is called Sono-elastography. It gives both qualitative and quantitative distribution of biological tissue strains and elasticity, and finds application in various clinical settings. There are two major applications Strain or Quasi-static elastography (QSE): This involves physical compression and displacement of tissues by the sonographer, which in turn induces a slow mechanical stress (strain) on tissues [15].

Both quantitative and qualitative assessment and comparison of the resulting stress is performed for tissues at rest and under compression. In order words the degree of stiffness, which is indicated by the range of tissue displacement is estimated. The degree of stiffness is represented quantitatively by a value and qualitatively in a color scale/mosaic that identifies the "softest" and "hardest" tissue areas. Strain sono-elastography provides a color map of tissue elasticity that is superimposed on the real-time greyscale ultrasound image. The stiffer the tissue, the more likelihood of being malignant. Consequently, in the breast, invasive cancers present as areas of higher stiffness compared to benign or normal tissues. A number of scoring systems have been developed to compare the presence, size and distribution of areas of elasticity within the supposed abnormality seen on a gray-scale image. This method appear to be more effective for superficially located structures such as breast and soft tissue masses. Shear wave elastography: This is a new method which combines the radiation force induced in a tissue by an ultrasonic beam and an ultrafast or supersonic imaging sequence which synchronizes the real- time propagation of the resulting shear waves. Typically, Shear waves cause particulate moves recorded with high-frequency imaging (5000 to 30,000 Hz), from which the system calculates color shades or elastograms in real-time (quantitative analysis).

This shear wave velocity enables the production of a two-dimensional map of shear elasticity. The technique is performed using a conventional linear array or special matrix probes. The effectiveness of shear wave elastography stems from the fact that the radiation force is automatically generated by the probe rather than the strain induced by an operator in conventional sono-elastography. Consequently, shear wave elastography is more reproducible than conventional or quasi-static elastography. Once an area has been mapped out by the cursor as region of interest (ROI), the values representing the mean and maximum stiffness are produced. The region corresponding to areas of stiffness can thus be mapped in a fairly reproducible, and quantitative manner. Benign lesions tend to be soft, while malignant lesions are generally stiffer. Applications include assessment of the degree of hepatic fibrosis and characterization of liver lesions, kidney, breast masses, prostate cancer detection, thyroid lesions and imaging of tendons.

6. Doppler studies

The application of Doppler principles in ultrasound imaging has a long history. Its use in the demonstration of blood vessels and patterns of flow have been copiously reported. Consequently, Doppler studies finds extensive clinical use in assessment of pregnancies, gynecology, cardio-vascular system, neonatalogy, surgery and small parts. The question of whether flow exists or not in a lesion is an important tool in resolving Dilemmas and recognizing or characterizing disease processes. It must be recognized that the increased use of ultrasound in musculo-skeletal imaging relate to the capability and ease of using real-time Doppler US [15]. The amount of flow in the tissue under investigation can be compared with the normal to make diagnosis easy. Doppler is particularly useful when evaluating tumor masses, inflammatory changes related to the joints, tendinopathies and some forms of neuropathies. It is also important when differentiating a ganglionic lesion from sarcoma, and in synovitis [15, 16]. The need to differentiate between acute synovitis (pannus) and chronic fibrotic synovium, is made possible by the demonstration of increased blood flow in the former. In fact, the presence of increased blood flow which is present in proliferating pannus fairly correlates with active joint destruction and symptom development. Consequently, ultrasound can make valuable judgment about the prognosis of active sinovitis and pathological sequel of aggressive and destructive changes in the joint. The deployment of Superb Microvascular Imaging in current studies has improved the resolution and sensitivity compared to conventional methods such as Power Doppler. It is known that superb microvascular Doppler technology allows the operator to detect low-grade inflammation, which was hitherto impossible with Power Doppler. The consequence of early detection of active inflammation, is the prospect of early intervention and impact on treatment outcomes [17].

7. Ultrafast Doppler ultrasound

There is an increasing interest in studying the function of human brain using neuro-imaging techniques [18]. In particular, ultrasonic waves which are transmitted at extremely high or ultrafast frame rates, have shown promise in detecting blood flow signals in very small vessels such as those that perfuse the brain [18]. This has been experimented in rodents with advantages of high spatial and temporal resolution, improved penetration and ability to detect microvascular changes associated with brain functions [18].

The advantages are further enhanced due to its portability and possibility of bedside use. Over the past one decade, bold attempts at applying the technique in preclinical imaging, creates room for wider possibilities in neonates, during operative surgery, or better still, the development of non-invasive brain machine interfaces [19]. The clinical application of this technique opens a new vista in the understanding of brain hemodynamics, changes following brain insult, and options for preserving neurological function [18, 19].

8. Conclusion

Refinements in technology continue to expand the capabilities and application of medical ultrasound in many clinical frontiers. One of the areas that has received significant acceptance is in its application to musculoskeletal and Neuro vascular disorders. This has further brought together a variety of clinical specialties such as orthopedics, vascular surgery, podiatry and physical therapy and rehabilitation medicine. The improvement in probe technology has allowed the development of ultra-fast high frequencies, with amazing results in spatial resolution, finer details, increased sensitivity and accessibility to obscure locations. The challenges of operator dependence and lack of standardized protocols have gradually been addressed due to increasing experience and applications by imaging experts [20].

Deployment of Doppler techniques such as Super micro vascular imaging, elastography, ultrafast Doppler and skilled maneuvers allow distinctive visualization of tissues such as joint capsular ligaments, tendons retinacula, fasciae and nerves all of which involve tiny mesenchymal structures whose diameters are in fractions of millimeters [11]. One more critical area of application is in the diagnostic evaluation of obscure masses [21]. These are essentially lesions in locations where conventional imaging modalities are less effective due to poor access. Such lesions include the perineum, vulva/labial regions, skin surfaces, abdominal walls and scalp [21]. The result is better diagnosis, improvement in patient navigation, quicker and easier treatment, less hospital stay, lower cost of health care and better prognosis. It is obvious that the future continues to hold better prospect for the ultrasound imaging of musculoskeletal systems.

Author details

Felix Okechukwu Erondu[1,2]

1 Department of Radiography and Radiation Sciences, College of Medicine and Health Sciences, Gregory University, Uturu, Abia State, Nigeria

2 Clinical Imaging, Image Diagnostics, Nigeria

*Address all correspondence to: okerons@yahoo.com

References

[1] Lawande AD, Warrier SS, Joshi MS. Role of ultrasound in evaluation of peripheral nerves. Indian Journal of Radiology and Imaging. 2014;**24**(3):254-258. DOI: 10.4103/0971-3026.137037

[2] Walker FO, Cartwright MS, Wiesler ER, Caress J. Ultrasound of nerve and muscle. Clinical Neurophysiology. 2004;**115**(3):495-507

[3] Romero-Morales C, Bravo-Aguilar M, Ruiz-Ruiz B, Almazán-Polo J, López-López D, Blanco-Morales M, et al. Current advances and research in ultrasound imaging to the assessment and management of musculoskeletal disorders. Disease-a-Month. 2021;**67**(3)

[4] Hodgson RJ, O'Connor PJ, Grainger AJ. Tendon and ligament imaging. The British Journal of Radiology. 2012;**85**(1016):1157-1172. DOI: 10.1259/bjr/34786470

[5] Fullerton GD, Rahal A. Collagen structure: the molecular source of the tendon magic angle effect. Journal of Magnetic Resonance Imaging. 2007;**25**:345-361

[6] Bruno F, Palumbo P, Arrigoni F, et al. Advanced diagnostic imaging and intervention in tendon diseases. Acta Biomed. 2020;**91**(8-S):98-106. DOI: 10.23750/abm.v91i8-S.10007

[7] De Filippo M, Pesce A, Barile A, et al. Imaging of postoperative shoulder instability. Musculoskeletal Surgery. 2017;**101**:15-22

[8] Barile A, Bruno F, Arrigoni F, et al. Emergency and trauma of the ankle. Seminars in Musculoskeletal Radiology. 2017;**21**:282-289

[9] Barile A, Bruno F, Mariani S, et al. Follow-up of surgical and minimally invasive treatment of Achilles tendon pathology: A brief diagnostic imaging review. Musculoskeletal Surgery. 2017;**101**:51-61

[10] Di Pietto F, Chianca V, de Ritis R, et al. Postoperative imaging in arthroscopic hip surgery. Musculoskeletal Surgery. 2017;**101**:43-49

[11] van Holsbeeck M, Soliman S, Van Kerkhove F, Craig J. Advanced musculoskeletal ultrasound techniques: What are the applications? American Journal of Roentgenology. 2021;**216**(2): 436-445

[12] Carrol AS, Simon NG. Current and future applications of ultrasound imaging in peripheral nerve disorders. World Journal of Radiology. 2020;**12**(6): 101-129. DOI: 10.4329/wjr.v12.i6.101

[13] Telleman JA, Grimm A, Goedee S, Visser LH, Zaidman CM. Nerve ultrasound in polyneuropathies. Muscle & Nerve. 2018;**57**:716-728

[14] Borire AA, Visser LH, Padua L, Colebatch JG, Huynh W, Simon NG, et al. Utility of maximum perfusion intensity as an ultrasonographic marker of intraneural blood flow. Muscle & Nerve. 2017;**55**:77-83

[15] Babaei-Ghazani A, Majdalani C-E, Luong DH, Front ABG. Sonoelastography of the shoulder: A narrative review. Frontiers in Rehabilitation Sciences. 2021;**2**(4):25. DOI: 10.3389/fresc.2021.704725

[16] Yokota K, Tsuzuki Wada T, Akiyama Y, Mimura T. Detection of synovial inflammation in rheumatic diseases using superb microvascular imaging: comparison with conventional power Doppler imaging. Modern Rheumatology. 2018;**28**:327-333

[17] Lim AKP, Satchithananda K, Dick EA, Abraham S, Cosgrove DO. Microflow imaging: New Doppler

technology to detect low-grade inflammation in patients with arthritis. European Radiology. 2018;**28**:1046-1053

[18] Demené C, Mairesse J, Baranger J, Tanter M, Baud O. Ultrafast Doppler for neonatal brain imaging. NeuroImage. 2019;**185**:851-856. DOI: 10.1016/j.neuroimage.2018.04.016

[19] Deffieux T, Demené C, Tanter M. Functional ultrasound imaging: A new imaging modality for neuroscience. Neuroscience. 2021;(474):110-121. DOI: 10.1016/j.neuroscience.2021.03.005

[20] Nazarian LN. The top 10 reasons musculoskeletal sonography is an important complementary or alternative technique to MRI. AJR. 2008;**190**: 1621-1626

[21] Erondu OF, Benson S, Ohuegbe I. Ultrasound as a convenient tool in the assessment of masses in obscure locations. Journal of Medicine and Medical Sciences. 2019;**10**(2):98

Chapter 5

Musculoskeletal and Nerve Ultrasonography

Stefan Cristian Dinescu, Razvan Adrian Ionescu, Horatiu Valeriu Popoviciu, Claudiu Avram and Florentin Ananu Vreju

Abstract

Musculoskeletal ultrasound had gained more and more importance lately and there is no doubt now about its role in the diagnosis and management of rheumatic diseases such as rheumatoid arthritis, spondyloarthritis, osteoarthritis and crystal related arthropathies. We can say that now, US is a widely available, non-invasive, and cost-effective technique suitable for the evaluation of the articular and periarticular structures, such as joints, tendons, muscles, ligaments, and bursa. The real-time capabilities of the US allow continuous observation of those structures during movement and of the needle placement during musculoskeletal interventions. More than this, recently, ultrasonography (US) has gained its rights in the evaluation of Sjogren syndrome and giant cell arteritis. Thus, US can detect changes secondary to both inflammatory joint diseases, like synovitis, tenosynovitis or enthesitis, and to degenerative disease, like osteophytes or tendinosis. US can identify calcium pyrophosphate and urate deposits at the level of the cartilage and tendons and to recognize the changes at the level of the salivary glands in the context of the Sjogren's syndrome and the ones at the level of the temporal artery, secondary to giant cell arteritis.

Keywords: rheumatology ultrasound, musculoskeletal, synovitis, enthesitis, nerve

1. Introduction

Ultrasonography (US) has become an integral part of the clinical rheumatology practice. It provides relevant information in many aspects of patient management, both diagnostic and therapeutic. It is a safe, non-invasive and readily accessible imaging modality, with a lack of contraindications. In this respect, US carries significant advantages over other imaging tests, such as CT or MRI. Musculoskeletal ultrasound provides the physician with a real-time evaluation, allows for a dynamic view of target areas and simultaneous scanning of multiple anatomical structures. It is fairly easy to apply imaging techniques, although it requires a prolonged period of training to achieve expert-level assessments. Musculoskeletal ultrasound (MSUS) allows for a fast examination of small and large joints and can guide further diagnostic tests. One of the most important benefits of MSUS is early diagnosis of articular and periarticular inflammation; this is especially the case in rheumatoid arthritis and psoriatic arthritis where diagnostic delay from symptom onset can lead to significant structural progression and poor outcomes. US evaluation is included in the EULAR (European League Against Rheumatism) recommendations for use of imaging in disease management for both RA and Spondyloarthritis (SpA) [1, 2]. Also, standardization of US procedure is provided through the EULAR standardized procedures for US imaging [3] and OMERACT (Outcome Measures in Rheumatoid Arthritis Clinical Trials) definitions of US pathology [4]. Apart from inflammatory and degenerative joint disease, US can also aid the rheumatologist in the diagnosis and management of connective tissue diseases such as systemic scleroderma, Sjögren's syndrome or vasculitis [5–7].

2. Principles of ultrasound examination in rheumatology

Ultrasonography enables detailed examination of anatomical structures, periarticular soft tissue and also blood flow using Doppler modalities. The 2017 EULAR standardized procedures for US [3] recommend the use of high-resolution linear transducers with a working frequency between 6 and 14 MHz for deeper structures and a frequency of ≥15 MHz for superficial areas. Probe compression can be used to distinguish compressible from non-compressible tissue, but should be avoided when examining blood flow. Images acquired in the long axis should be oriented with the proximal aspect to the left of the screen, while in the short axis, the structures of interest will be aligned just as the examiner is looking at the patient.

US evaluation can assess bone surface, cartilage, tendons, ligaments, synovial proliferation and bursal effusions. Additionally, soft tissue US will include examination of blood vessels, skin, adipose tissue, peripheral nerves for entrapment or tumors (**Figure 1**) and muscles that can be scanned for inflammation, lesions or fluid collections [8].

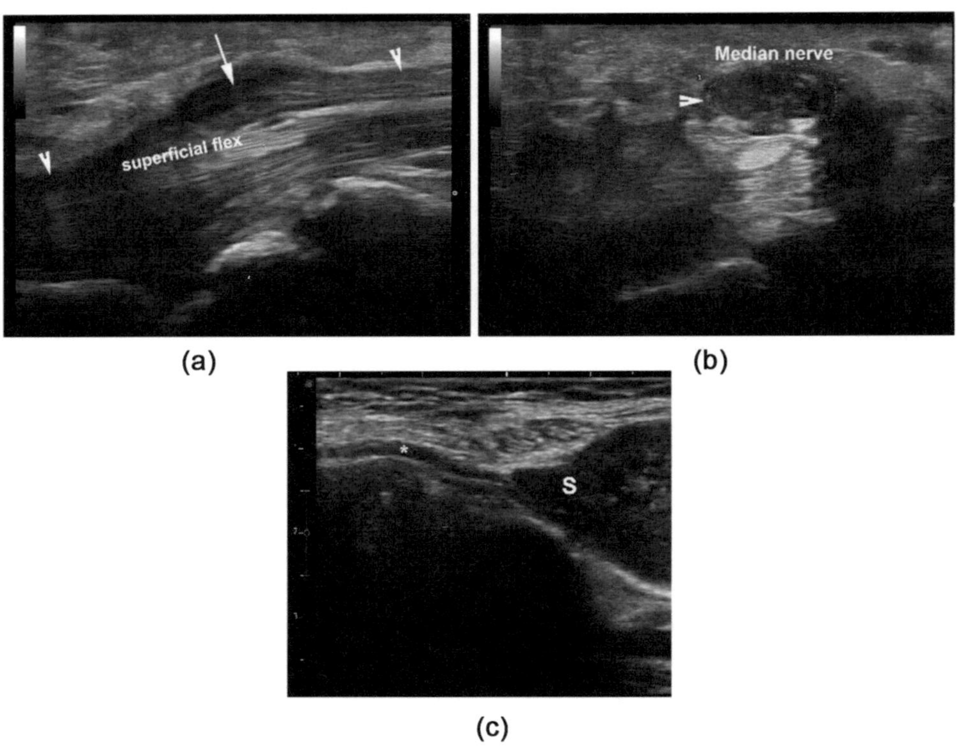

Figure 1.
Ultrasound GS images of a median nerve neuroma (a – Longitudinal, b - transverse) and a peroneal schwannoma (c - longitudinal). Arrowhead – Median nerve, arrow – Neuroma, asterisk – Peroneal nerve, S – Schwannoma.

The study of blood flow is important in detecting inflammatory activity and this can be performed using color Doppler or power Doppler modalities [9]. Because in the musculoskeletal US, the blood flow is very slow in the small new vessels formed by inflammatory angiogenesis, the pulse repetition frequency used is low, under 1KHz. Nevertheless, some small vessel blood flow is difficult to detect because the signal intensity can be lower than movement artifacts and will be filtered out [10].

Ultrasonography is examiner-dependent, thus a good clinical experience, knowledge of anatomy, good image acquisition and reading of the ultrasound images, together with pitfalls recognition are needed requirements for a quality examination. The OMERACT task-force group has developed standardized definitions to promote uniformity between US examiners' reports (see **Table 1**).

Additional information during US imaging can be obtained through sonoelastography and contrast-enhanced ultrasonography (CEUS) [11–15]. These two US techniques have been studied and proven their usefulness in certain rheumatic diseases, but nevertheless, they are not so widely used as conventional gray scale (GS) and Doppler modalities. Sonoelastography is used for measuring and quantifying tissue stiffness. This can be applied in various situations such as tendon lesions, myositis, and analysis of soft tissue formations such as gout tophi or rheumatoid nodules [16, 17]. Also, promising results are seen in studies of systemic scleroderma, where skin involvement is correlated with loss of dermal elasticity [5]. CEUS can assess joint inflammation and provides a view of the exact vascular patterns, which can also be visible in inflamed sacroiliac joints [10, 18]. Some studies report the superiority of CEUS compared to power Doppler US in detecting synovial hypervascularity [14, 15]. Compared to the known risks of using contrast agents in MRI and CT, contrast agents used in CEUS have no proof of significant side-effects.

Further use of ultrasonography in rheumatology practice resides in the ability to guide local procedures. These include synovial fluid aspiration, therapeutic injection, nerve blocks or soft tissue biopsy [19]. US guided infiltrations have proven to significantly increase the accuracy of medication placement when compared to infiltration guided by anatomical landmarks [20]. This is also the case in aspiration of small fluid effusions or fluid cavities which have multiple septa. Besides the accuracy of therapy injection, US-guided procedures have a reduced risk of damaging nearby nerves, tendons or blood vessels.

Bone Erosion	A step-down intraarticular discontinuity of the bone surface is visible in 2 perpendicular planes.
Synovial Fluid	Abnormal displaceable and compressible, hypoechoic or anechoic (in comparison to subdermal fat) intraarticular material, that does not exhibit Doppler signal. To note that sometimes it may be isoechoic or hyperechoic
Synovial Hypertrophy	Abnormal non-displaceable, but poorly compressible, hypoechoic intraarticular tissue (relative to subdermal fat), that may sometimes be isoechoic or hyperechoic. The Doppler signal might be present.
Tenosynovitis	The thickened tendon sheath, with hypoechoic or anechoic material inside, which is seen in 2 perpendicular planes, and which may exhibit Doppler signal. Also, fluid might be present.
Enthesopathy	Thickened tendon or ligament at its bony attachment, with loss of normal fibrillar architecture, looking abnormally hypoechoic (may contain calcifications, seen as hyperechoic foci and/or bony changes including enthesophytes, erosions, or irregularity), identified in 2 perpendicular planes. It may exhibit a Doppler signal.

Table 1.
OMERACT definitions of ultrasound lesions [4].

Despite being highly sensitive to inflammatory features, sometimes US cannot discriminate between underlying diseases, especially when suspecting septic arthritis. Here, arthrocentesis can aid the diagnosis through fluid analysis in Gram stain, culture, as well as polarized microscopy.

3. Pathology

3.1 Rheumatoid arthritis

Musculoskeletal ultrasound is frequently used in clinical practice when approaching a patient with joint pain or during the management of a patient with an established diagnosis of RA. US examination can provide valuable information and is often essential for differential diagnosis. Gutierez et al. established in a study on 204 patients with undifferentiated arthritis that US can help fulfill the ACR 2010 criteria and led to a modified diagnosis in 42.1% of cases [21]. This is very insightful because it points out to a significant proportion of patients, mainly seronegative cases with limited joint involvement that could be underdiagnosed within the first months from symptom onset. The 2013 EULAR recommendations for imaging in RA have taken this into account and highlighted the importance of early detection of inflammation and structural damage in patients with arthritis in at least one joint [1]. 9 out of 10 recommendations included the use of ultrasound. This stands for the potential benefit of US in the whole disease spectrum: detection of subclinical inflammation, prediction of progression, differential diagnosis and disease monitoring [22, 23].

The US features seen in RA include: synovial proliferation, joint effusion, cortical bone erosions (**Figure 2c** and **d**) and tenosynovitis. Among these, the presence of erosions and synovial proliferation are considered more specific (**Figure 2**). Moreover, synovial thickening with an increased power Doppler signal can differentiate between active and inactive inflammation [24]. The presence of active inflammation on US and bone marrow edema on MRI can predict risk for radiological progression even in asymptomatic joints. The potential for predicting erosive damage has also been proven for features of tenosynovitis [25].

There is significant evidence related to residual inflammation in clinical remission which in this case could be considered an unstable remission [26]. This can predict a disease flare or structural damage in asymptomatic cases within one year [27].

A more accurate evaluation of inflammatory features detected in RA patients will include a semi-quantified scoring system. This has proven to be correlated with disease activity and can aid the clinician in follow-up visits. The OMERACT study group provided grading systems for synovitis in both gray scale and Doppler mode [4] (see **Table 2**). In 2017, the EULAR-OMERACT study group integrated them into a combined scoring system for synovitis (see **Table 3**) [28].

For practical reasons, a physician should limit the number of joints included in one ultrasound examination. The exact number of joints that should be assessed will certainly depend on clinical presentation, but some studies have provided guidance for a more efficient imaging session. Naredo and colleagues proposed the examination of 12 joints using power Doppler which can provide an overall assessment of joint inflammation. The sites included bilateral wrists, second and third MCPs, and second and third PIPs of hands and knee joints [30]. In 2009, Backhaus and colleagues proposed a more limited number of joints which formed the German US7 score. This score included the wrists, II and III MCPs and PIPs, II and V MTPs joints of the clinically dominant hand and foot [31].

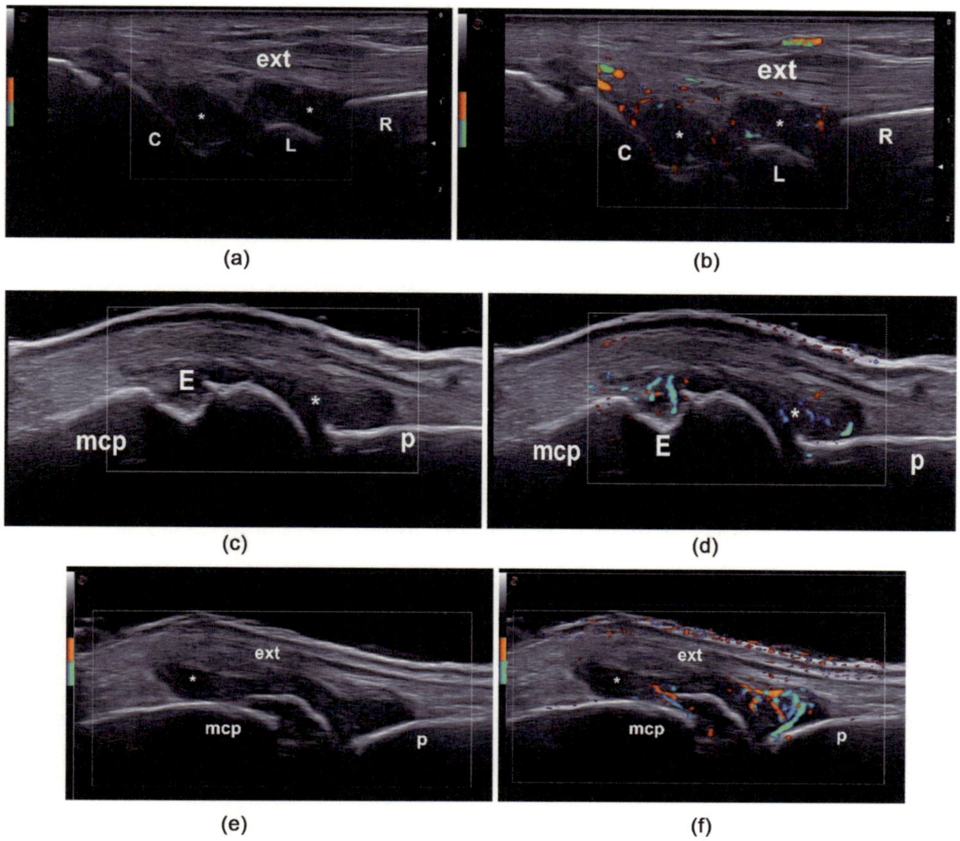

Figure 2.
Synovitis in GS (left images) and with power Doppler (right images) at the level of the wrist (a) and metacarpophalangeal joints (c-f). e – Erosions, ext. – Extensor tendons, mcp - metacarpal bone, p – Phalanx, asterisk – Synovitis.

GS	Grade 0: Normal joint (no synovial hypertrophy, no joint effusion)
	Grade 1: Minimal synovitis (minimal synovial hypertrophy, with or without minimal joint effusion)
	Grade 2: Moderate synovitis (moderate synovial hypertrophy, with or without minimal or moderate joint effusion)
	Grade 3: Severe synovitis (severe synovial hypertrophy, with or without severe joint effusion)
Power-Doppler	Grade 0: No vessels in the synovial membrane
	Grade 1: Up to 3 single color spots or 1 confluent spot plus other up to 2 single spots
	Grade 2: Doppler signal in <50% of the synovium
	Grade 3: Doppler signal in >50% of the synovium

Table 2.
OMERACT scoring system for synovitis [4].

Musculoskeletal ultrasound has proved a strong correlation with other disease activity markers such as the DAS28 score, ESR or CRP levels [32]. Nevertheless, detection of US inflammation is still possible in the context of DAS28 remission and this could influence treatment decisions [12]. US features are sensible to RA-specific

Grade 0: Normal joint	No synovial hypertrophy (SH) in GS and no PD signal (within the synovium)
Grade 1: Minimal synovitis	Grade 1 SH in GS and ≤ Grade 1 PD signal
Grade 2: Moderate synovitis	Grade 2 GS synovial hypertrophy and ≤ Grade 2 PD signal or Grade 1 SH in GS and a Grade 2 PD signal
Grade 3: Severe synovitis	GS grade 3 SH and ≤ Grade 3 PD signal or Grade 1 or 2 synovial hypertrophy in GS and a Grade 3 PD signal

SH – synovial hypertrophy; PD – power Doppler.
In addition, erosive changes have also been integrated into a 0–3 scale for each individual erosion, based on the maximum length. The scoring ultrasound structural erosion (ScUSSe) system is used as follows: 0 = no erosion, 1 = <2 mm, 2 = 2–3 mm, 3 = >3 mm [29].

Table 3.
EULAR-OMERACT combined scoring system for synovitis [28].

therapies and this has also been proven for local intraarticular steroid injections [24]. Thus, ultrasound is a helpful tool for monitoring treatment response.

3.2 Spondyloarthritis

Imaging tests commonly used in patients with axial spondyloarthritis are based mainly on the detection of sacroiliitis through conventional radiology or MRI. The use of ultrasound in SpA patients becomes relevant in peripheral involvement and especially in patients with psoriatic arthritis (PsA). US features seen in SpA patients include: arthritis, tenosynovitis, enthesitis and dactylitis. As in RA, Doppler mode is useful to confirm active inflammation in the articular and periarticular structures. Compared to RA, tenosynovitis (**Figure 3**) is more prevalent, while enthesitis and dactylitis are considered specific features of SpA.

The presence of the lesions on US can help differentiate PsA from early RA. Moreover, psoriatic arthritis patients have proven some other discriminative

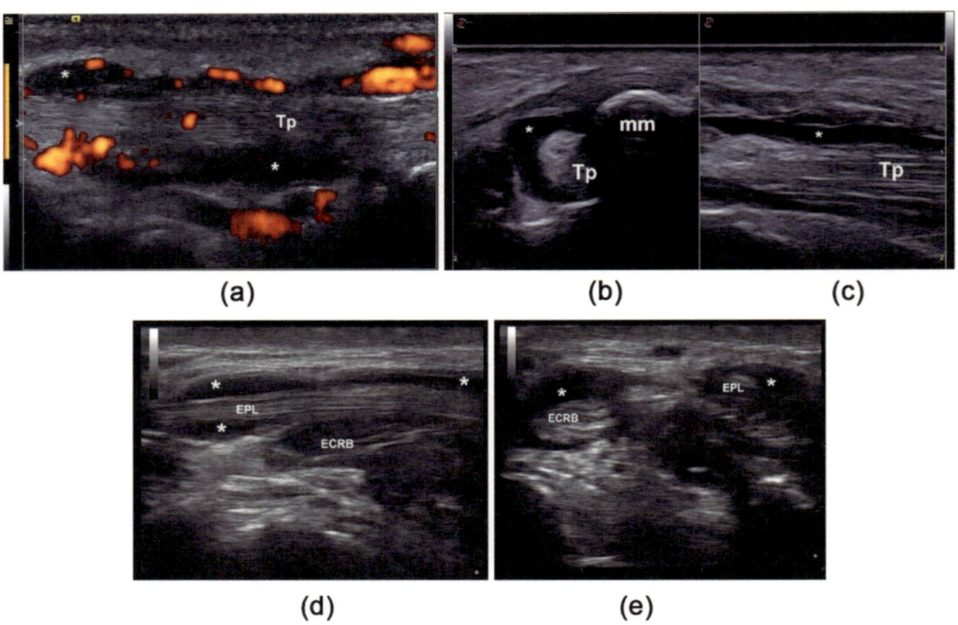

Figure 3.
Ultrasonography of the tibialis posterior (Tp) tenosynovitis (a-c, asterisk) and at the level of extensor carpi radialis brevis (ECRB) and extensor pollicis longus (EPL). mm – Medial malleolus.

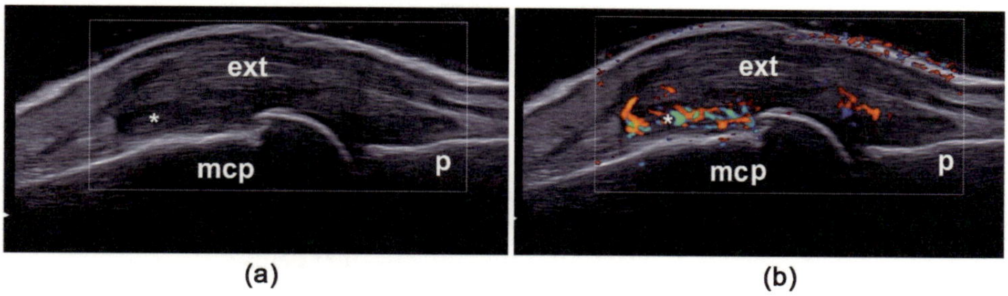

Figure 4.
Ultrasonography of the metacarpophalangeal joints in GS mode (left) and power Doppler (right), with periextensor tendon inflammation (PTI pattern - asterisk). mcp – Metacarpal bone, p – Phalanx, ext. – Extensor tendon.

features such as peritendon extensor digitorum tendon inflammation (**Figure 4**) and central slip enthesitis at the PIP joints [33].

The 2015 EULAR recommendations for the use of imaging in the diagnosis and management of SpA [2] have included ultrasound in three recommendations for peripheral SpA regarding diagnosis, monitoring activity and monitoring structural changes, as follows:

- *Recommendation 2 for peripheral SpA*

  Peripheral arthritis, tenosynovitis and bursitis may be **detected** by **US** or MRI. Furthermore, those imaging techniques may be used to detect peripheral enthesitis, which might support the **diagnosis** of SpA.

- *Recommendation 5 for peripheral SpA*

  US with high-frequency color or power Doppler and MRI may be used to **monitor disease activity** in peripheral SpA, the decision on when to repeat US/MRI depending on the clinical circumstances.

- *Recommendation 6 for peripheral SpA*

  When the clinical scenario requires monitoring of structural damage in peripheral SpA, MRI and/or **US might provide additional information,** besides conventional radiography.

The OMERACT Ultrasound Task Force published in 2013 a consensus regarding ultrasound score for tenosynovitis (see **Table 4**). A four grade-semiquantitative scoring system is proposed for both gray-scale (grade 0, normal; grade 1, minimal;

grade 0	no Doppler signal
grade 1	focal Doppler signal within the widened synovial sheath, identified in two perpendicular planes, excluding normal feeding vessels
grade 2	multifocal Doppler signal within the widened synovial sheath, seen in two perpendicular planes, excluding normal feeding vessels
grade 3	diffuse Doppler signal inside the widened synovial sheath, seen in two perpendicular planes, excluding normal feeding vessels

Table 4.
OMERACT ultrasound task force scoring system for tenosynovitis using Doppler mode [30].

grade 2, moderate; grade 3, severe) and Doppler mode (grade 0, no Doppler signal; grade 1, minimal; grade 2, moderate; grade 3, severe) [30].

Enthesitis is broadly defined as inflammation of the fibrocartilaginous tissue located at the insertion points of tendons (**Figure 5**), ligaments and the joint capsule on bone surface. US features related to enthesitis that have met the 2018 OMERACT consensus [34] include: hypoechogenicity, increased thickness of enthesis, erosions and calcifications/enthesophytes and Doppler signal at insertion. Increased tendon thickness, hypoechogenicity and shadowing of the fibrillar pattern are seen in earlier phases of enthesitis, while cortical bone changes, in the form of erosions and enthesophytes, are related to later stages [35]. Moreover, lesions should be restricted to <2 mm from cortical bone [34]. Nevertheless, distinguishing physiologic entheseal changes in active adults from disease-related lesions may be difficult. Also, lower extremity entheses are prone to mechanical loading, especially in obese patients [36].

When examining enthesis sites for inflammation, a selective approach is required. This will take into account the more accessible areas, present symptoms and potential confounding factors. Various research groups have proposed different sets of enthesis scoring systems. These include the: GUESS - Glasgow Ultrasound Enthesitis Score [37], MASEI - Madrid Sonography Enthesitis Index [38], GRAPPA US - proposed entheseal sites by the GRAPPA Ultrasound Working Group [39] and OMERACT US - proposed entheseal sites by the OMERACT Ultrasound Enthesitis Working Group [34].

New research revealed other areas in which we can find structures that can be assimilated to enthesis. Thus, we can consider as functional enthesis the areas of tendons or ligaments that are wrapped around by pulleys, without being attached to them and as articular fibrocartilaginous entheses, the synovial joints lined with fibrocartilage [40]. Inflammation of those entheses can be identified by US and can explain pain in specific areas.

Dactylitis, one of the more complex inflammatory lesions seen in SpA, is a pandigital disease that involves joint arthritis, tenosynovitis of the flexors, enthesitis of the

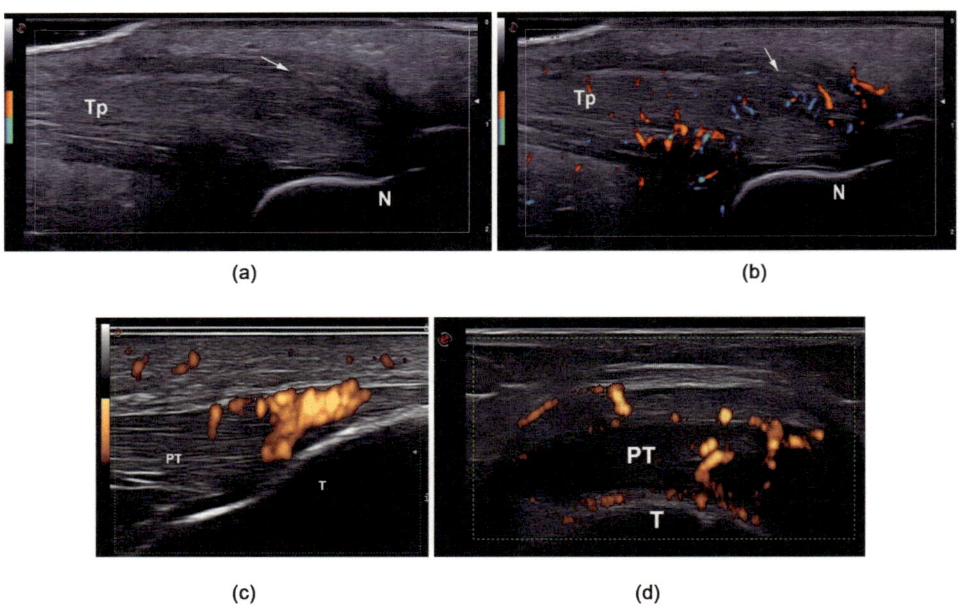

Figure 5.
Ultrasonography of the tibialis posterior (a, b – Longitudinal aspect) (Tp) enthesitis (arrow) at the level of the navicular tuberosity (N) in GS (left) and power Doppler modes (right) and enthesitis of the patellar tendon (c – longitudinal, d – transverse). PT – Patellar tendon, T – tibia.

superficial flexor of the finger, functional enthesitis, proximal to metacarpophalangeal joint (periextensor tendon inflammation) and soft tissue edema (**Figure 6**) [36, 41]. Of this spectrum of lesions, tenosynovitis (**Figure 5**) is considered the primary cause for the characteristic dactylitis or sausage-like appearance of the fingers. Flexor tenosynovitis and joint synovitis are the most frequent features seen in 90% of cases [11]. US lesions related to dactylitis evolve over time. Earlier phases are marked by tenosynovitis and lack of joint inflammation, while in later stages, joint synovitis is more prevalent in comparison to an absent or minimal tenosynovitis [42].

Dactylitis has a relevant role in the early diagnosis of PsA and has also been used as an outcome measure in clinical trials. This has prompted the development of sonographic scores for dactylitis, such as the DACTOS score. It is a composite score which includes the following: peritendinous inflammation of the extensors (PTI), evaluated in GS and PD at the MCP and PIP joints levels (with the maximum score of 4); soft tissue oedema; flexor tenosynovitis evaluated in GS and PD noted in the most severely affected area of the digit (with the maximum score of 6 for each); the combined score for synovitis (evaluated according to EULAR-OMERACT definitions) at the MCP, PIP, and DIP joints (maximum score of 9) [41]. DACTOS score is sensitive to treatment and correlates well with Leeds Dactylitis Index basic, as well as VAS for pain and functional impairment [43].

3.3 Crystal deposition disease

Gout and chondrocalcinosis are the two main forms of crystal deposition disease in which crystals of different compositions accumulate in the intraarticular space and periarticular soft tissue. In gout, raised uric acid levels in the serum to lead to deposition of monosodium urate (MSU) crystals. Chondrocalciosis, also called pseudogout, is characterized by the deposition of calcium pyrophosphate dihydrate (CPPD) crystals. Apart from the different chemical compositions, the both disorders have specific imaging features on ultrasound [17]. MSU crystals in gout generate a characteristic hyperechoic band on the cartilage surface [44], known as the "double contour sign" (**Figure 7**). The dynamic evaluation of the joint reveals the urate hyperechoic band moving together with the bone, thus confirming the belonging to the bone cartilage. This is observed in the majority of gout patients and is reversible with treatment.

MSU deposits can precipitate in the synovial membrane, in the joint cavity within synovial effusion (**Figure 8a–c**), in tendons, bursae and soft tissues. Gout tophi appear as a heterogeneous mass with intermittent hyperechoic foci and can

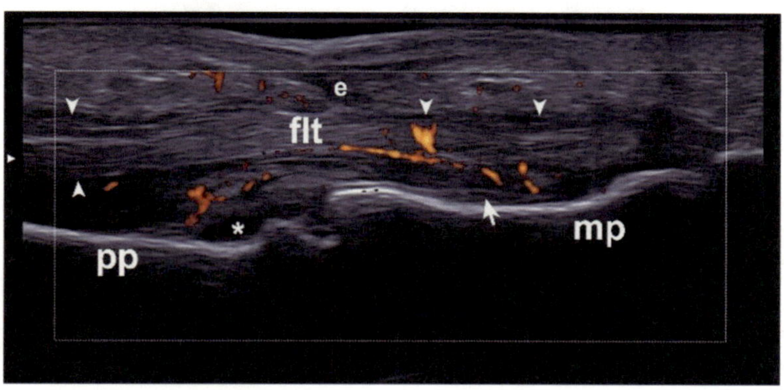

Figure 6.
Ultrasound image of a volar aspect of the finger, showing changes specific to dactylitis. pp – Proximal phalanx, mp – Medial phalanx, flt – Flexor tendon, asterisk – Synovitis, e - soft tissue oedema, arrow - enthesitis of the superficial flexor tendon, arrowheads – Flexor tenosynovitis.

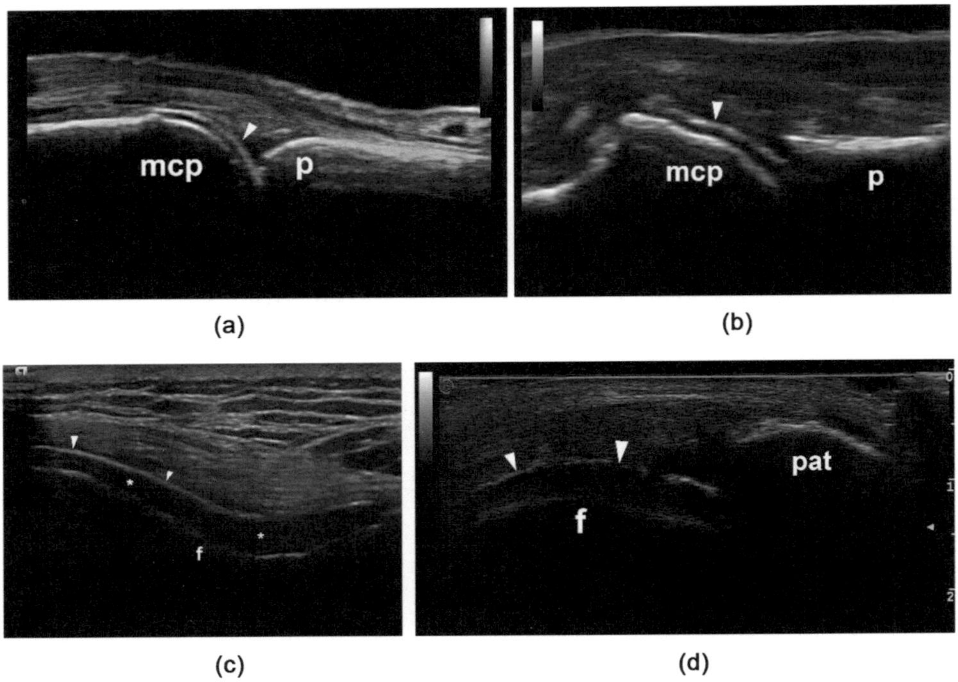

Figure 7.
"Double contour sign" (arrow head) in US of the metacarpophalangeal (a, b) and knee joints (c, d), in longitudinal (a, b, d) and transverse section (c). mcp – metacarpal bone, p – phalanx, f – femur, pat – patella, asterisk – hyalin cartilage.

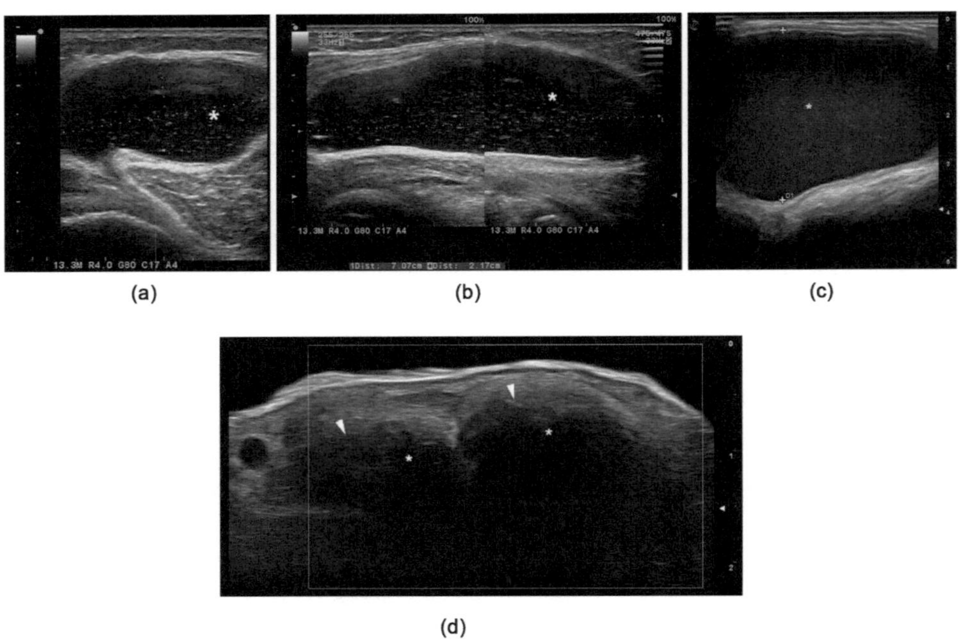

Figure 8.
a–c. Ultrasound images of gouty synovial effusion at the level of the posterior knee – Popliteal cyst (a - transverse, b - longitudinal) and of the olecranon bursa, with the aspect of the "snowstorm" (anechoic area with hyperechoic spots). d. Gouty tophus (arrowhead), with posterior acoustic shadowing (asterisk).

be distinguished from lipoma or rheumatoid nodules which are more hypoechoic and homogenous. Features of MSU crystal deposition inside tendons and joints and even tophi (**Figure 8d**) can be detected in the setting of asymptomatic

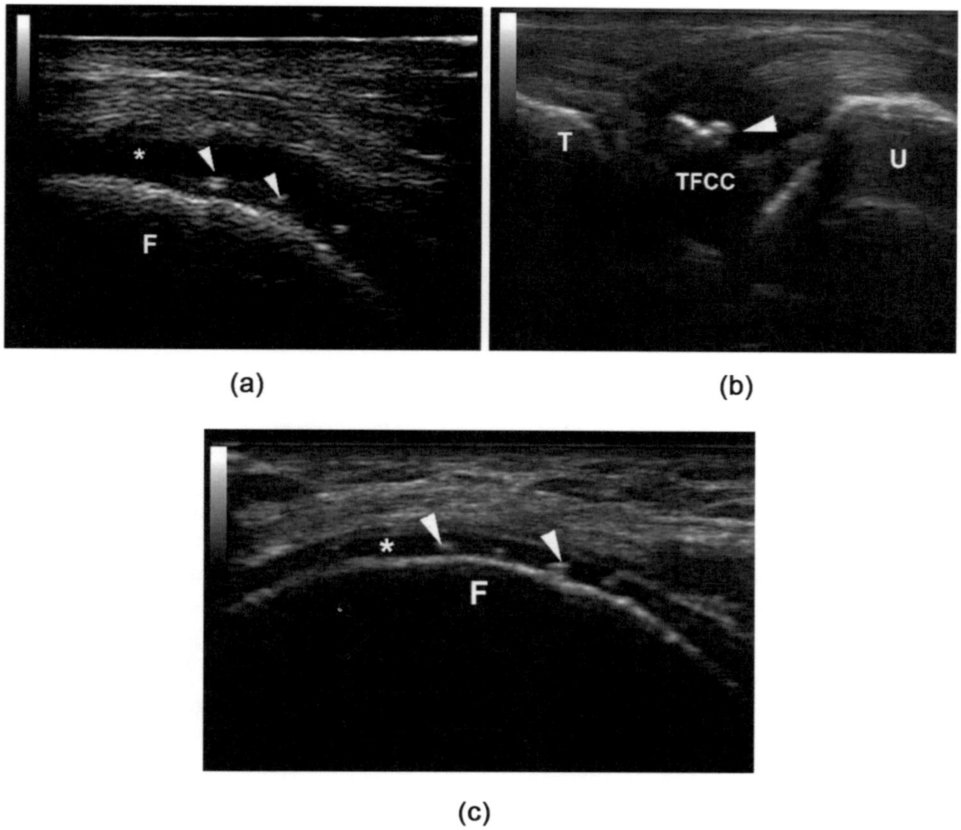

Figure 9.
Ultrasound images of calcium pyrophosphate deposits (arrowheads) in CPPD, inside the knee hyaline cartilage (a, c) and in the triangular fibrocartilage complex (b). F – Femur, TFCC - triangular fibrocartilage complex, asterisk – Hyaline cartilage.

hyperuricemia. EULAR and ACR recommendations support the use of ultrasound in gout and CPPD due to its high sensitivity and specificity [45–47]. The 2015 EULAR/ACR gout classification criteria recognize ultrasound and dual-energy computed tomography as the main imaging modalities used to accurately identify urate deposition [46].

The 2011 EULAR recommendations for calcium pyrophosphate deposition disease (CPPD) highlight the diagnostic potential of ultrasound with a high diagnosis likelihood ratio and possibly even better sensitivity than those of conventional x-rays [47]. The paper of Filippou demonstrated US to be an accurate tool for discriminating CPPD [48]. The OMERACT US group for CPPD has defined in 2017, the ultrasonographic characteristics of CPPD, in both joints and periarticular tissues [49, 50]. In contrast to gouty deposits appearance, at the surface of the cartilage, in CPPD the deposits are present inside the hyaline cartilage. The most important joints in which we can find CPPD deposits are the wrist (at the level of the triangular fibrocartilage), the knee (meniscus and hyaline cartilage) (**Figure 9**), acromioclavicular and hip joint [50].

3.4 Osteoarthritis

Features of degenerative joint disease are easily recognizable by ultrasound examination. Lesions related to osteoarthritis include varying degrees of cartilage damage and osteophyte formation. Although, conventional x-ray is also commonly used in osteoarthritis diagnosis, it can be fairly limited in earlier phases and lacks the capacity to directly visualize the articular hyaline cartilage. One of

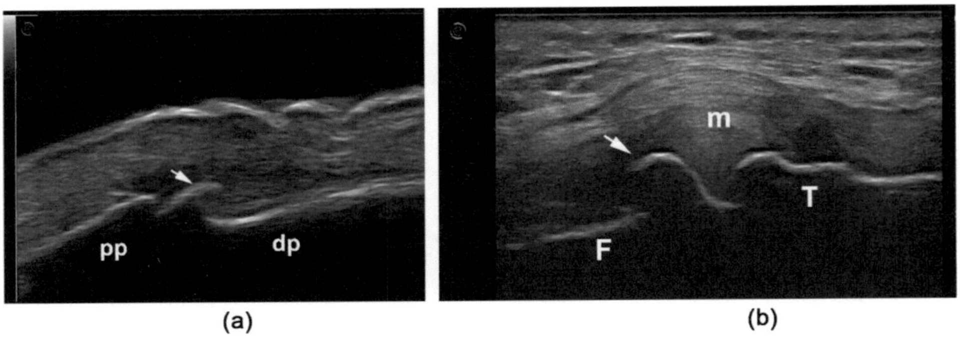

Figure 10.
Ultrasound images of step-up bony prominences, at the level of the interphalangeal (a) and femurotibial (b) joints, suggestive for osteophytes. pp – proximal phalanx, dp – distal phalanx, F – femur, T – tibia, m – meniscus, arrow - osteophyte.

the hallmarks of osteoarthritis US features is the diminished cartilage thickness. Normally, the hyaline cartilage appears as a well-defined anechoic band, due to increased water content, which lacks internal echoes [17]. US has proven to have higher sensitivity compared to conventional x-ray in the assessment of osteophytes and space narrowing. Early features of OA visible through US include: loss of the sharp contour, asymmetric thinning and changes in echogenicity of the cartilage matrix. Additionally, some forms of OA can display erosive and inflammatory changes [51]. Osteophytes are defined as step-up bony prominence seen in two perpendicular planes (**Figure 10**).

The presence of cortical bone irregularities and bony erosions can lead to difficulties in distinguishing osteophyte formations. Upon detection of osteophytes various scoring systems can be applied. This can be a simple semi-quantitative grading scale, as follows: 0 = No osteophyte, 1 = Marginal osteophyte, 2 = Medium osteophyte, 3 = Large osteophyte. Mortada and colleagues proposed a more detailed scoring system for the severity of knee osteoarthritis (see **Table 5**) [52].

The musculoskeletal US can also be applied for therapeutic purposes in degenerative diseases. Patients with OA can benefit from intra-articular infiltration with hyaluronic acid or glucocorticoid and this can be more accurately performed through ultrasound-guided injections. Besides the immediate release of synovial fluid visible during joint aspiration, inflammatory features have also proven to decrease posttreatment. Hence, ultrasound has become a useful tool in both local treatment and monitoring disease activity.

Grade 0		No osteophytes; regular end of femoral condyle without any projections.
Grade 1		Minor osteophyte; just a small projection from the femoral condyle.
Grade 2	2A	Small osteophytes; a projection from the femoral condyle that appears to have an inferior part in the joint space zone.
	2B	Large osteophyte appears to be separated from femoral condyle and to have an inferior part in joint space zone.
Grade 3		Large osteophyte appears to be separated from femoral condyle and to have an inferior part in joint space zone with small superior extension parallel to femoral bone.
Grade 4		Mainly superior osteophyte parallel to the femoral bone with or without an inferior part in joint space zone.

Table 5.
Ultrasonographic grading scale for severity of primary knee osteoarthritis by Mortada et al. [52].

3.5 Scleroderma

One of the most important clinical features of patients with systemic sclerosis (SSc) is the skin thickening. The extent of skin features in SSc is divided clinically into diffuse and limited involvement and is usually quantified using the Rodnan skin score. In addition to this, high-frequency ultrasound can also allow for a detailed assessment of skin involvement. The target measurement is the dermal thickness. For a correct assessment, the following interfaces need to be identified: surface–epidermis, epidermis–dermis and dermis–subcutis [53]. Skin features in SSc vary in time and this is detectable also through US. In the edematous phase, increased thickness associated with low echogenicity is seen due to water content. In time, fibrosis leads to increased echogenicity. Ultrasound measurements correlated well with histopathology, Rodnan skin score and EUSTAR disease activity index [5, 54]. Hongyan and colleagues defined an optimal cutoff point of 7.4 mm for skin thickness, with a sensitivity of 77.4% and specificity of 87.1% [54]. Quantitative studies of skin stiffness using sonoelastography yielded promising results. Research by Yang and colleagues indicates that Shear Wave Elastography can discriminate between SSc patients and controls (**Figure 11**), has good reliability and correlates well with skin thickness and modified Rodnan skin sore [55].

3.6 Sjögren's syndrome

Primary Sjögren's syndrome (pSS) is an autoimmune disease of the exocrine glands, which manifests mainly as hyposecretion of salivary and lacrimal glands. The diagnosis approach is generally focused on the detection of specific autoantibodies, positive ocular tests and findings of characteristic histopathological abnormalities. Sialography and scintigraphy are considered invasive and rarely used in everyday practice, while limited accessibility and the high cost of MRI also hinders its use. Studies on ultrasound have produced promising results for the assessment of major salivary glands (**Figure 12**) of pSS patients and offer a more accessible and less time-consuming alternative to other imaging tests. Still, the established

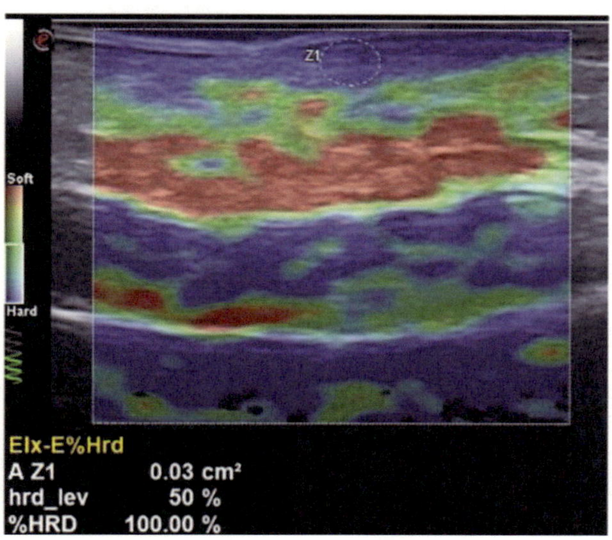

Figure 11.
Elastography of the finger volar aspect that shows the increased hardness of the epidermis and dermis, as shown by the blue color and the hardness percent.

diagnostic criteria developed up until now for pSS have not included ultrasonography as a recommended diagnostic tool.

The parotid and submandibular glands can be easily examined for certain structural abnormalities, such as: parenchymal inhomogeneity, hypo-anechoic or hyperechoic areas (**Figure 12b** and **c**) (produced by cysts or calcifications), surface irregularities and changes in glandular size, intra- or periglandular lymph nodes [56].

Additionally, the use of Doppler modes can identify glandular hypervascularization which has been consistently observed in pSS patients. In early phases, US is marked by an increase in glandular volume and high vascularity, while in later stages reduced volume and hypovascularization are characteristic [57]. Parenchymal inhomogeneity is the most recognizable term used in the development of numerous grading systems.

Research carried out by De Vita et al. [58], Hocevar et al. [59] and Salaffi et al. [60] provided some of the well-known semiquantitative scoring systems. All of these US scores proved high sensitivity and specificity for pSS. De Vita et al. developed a 0-3 scale for parenchymal inhomogeneity, while Hocevar et al. added 0-3 scales also for the number of hypoechogenic areas, hyperechogenic reflections and clearness of salivary gland border. Salaffi et al. proposed an extended 0-4 scale for parenchymal inhomogeneity which includes all of the features previously mentioned (see **Table 6**) [60].

Minor salivary gland biopsy remains the gold standard for diagnosis and is recommended in most patients with suspected pSS, especially in cases with positive autoantibodies. Studies evaluated the predictive value of salivary gland US for histopathology abnormalities. Miedany et al. [61] found a significant correlation between US score and histopathological score ($r = 0.82$). This supports the use of US when biopsy cannot be performed or in order to stratify the at-risk patients before ordering a biopsy.

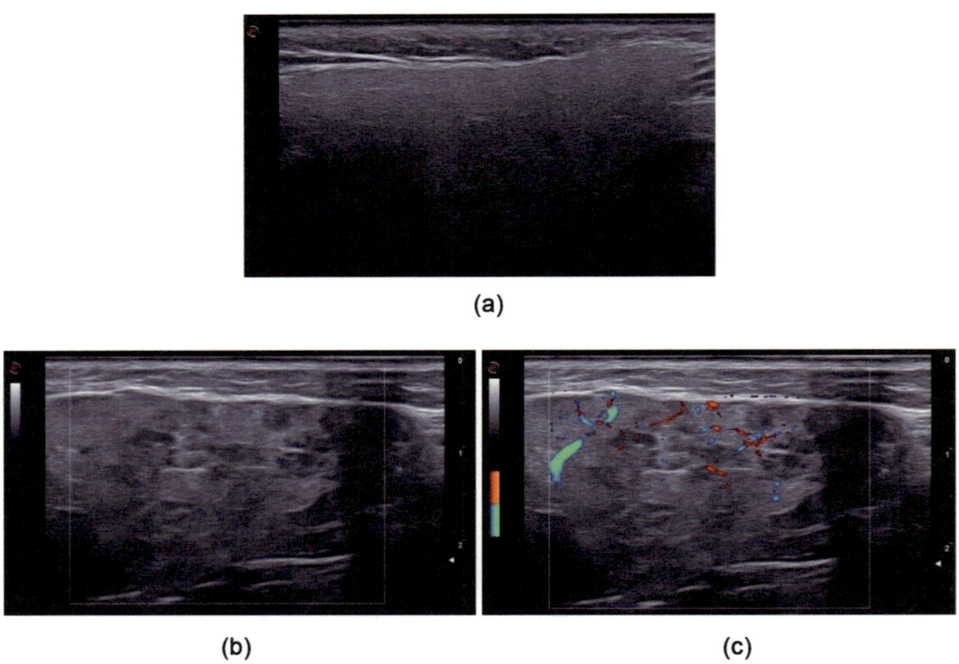

Figure 12.
a. Normal aspect of a parotid gland. b, c. Parotid gland US in GS (b) and PD (c) modes, with the inhomogeneous aspect, with multiple hypoechoic areas, suggestive for glandular inflammation.

Grade 0	normal US aspect of the glands
Grade 1	regular contour, small hypoechoic areas, without echogenic bands, normal or increased glandular volume (with mean values 20 + 3 mm for the parotids and 13 + 2 mm for the submandibular glands) and badly defined posterior border (definite echogenic border with respect to the neighboring structures)
Grade 2	regular contour, numerous dispersed hypoechogenic areas of variable size (<2 mm), without echogenic bands, normal or increased glandular volume and badly defined posterior border
Grade 3	irregular contour, multiple, moderate in size (2–6 mm), circumscribed or confluent hypoechogenic areas and/or multiple cysts, with echogenic bands, regular or decreased glandular volume and no visible posterior border
Grade 4	irregular contour, multiple, large (>6 mm), circumscribed or confluent hypoechogenic areas, and/or multiple cysts or multiple calcifications, with echogenic bands, resulting in severe change of the glandular architecture, decreased glandular volume and posterior glandular border not visible

Table 6.
Ultrasound semiquantitative scoring system for parenchymal inhomogeneity by Salaffi et al. [60].

3.7 Large vessel vasculitis

Ultrasound imaging can detect signs of arterial involvement in giant cell arteritis and Takayasu disease. The characteristic US features of large vessel vasculitis include the presence of a hypoechoic swollen artery wall which is surrounded by oedema, known as the halo sign (**Figure 13**).

The use of US has been studied more extensively in giant cell arteritis. Detection of the typical patchy inflammation seen in temporal arteritis can benefit greatly from ultrasound examination. Besides wall thickening, large vessel vasculitis can display lack of compressibility, stenosis and vessel occlusion [6]. Importantly, giant cell arteritis can spare the temporal arteries in some cases, and thus US examination should also include other large vessels such as the axillary or carotid arteries. The diagnostic value of US has been highlighted by its adoption in the 2018 Update of the EULAR recommendations for the management of large vessel vasculitis. Ultrasound examination is included in the imaging tests used to confirm the diagnosis when large vessel vasculitis is suspected [62].

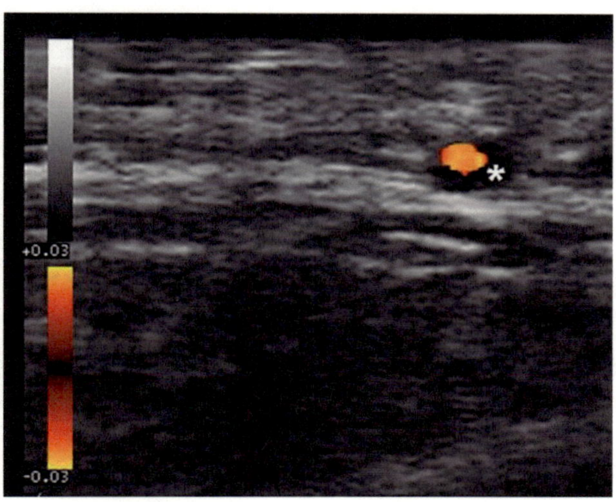

Figure 13.
Ultrasonography of the temporal artery showing a swollen hypoechoic wall – Halo sign (asterisk).

3.8 Muscular disease

Various muscle pathologies can be assessed using ultrasonography. It can detect partial and complete muscle ruptures, fluid collections, muscle infarctions or development of muscle tumors. Features of posttraumatic lesions vary by severity. Milder intensity trauma leads to interstitial hemorrhage which appears as poorly defined hyperechoic areas. In more severe trauma, an intramuscular hematoma can develop, and echogenicity will vary based on time of lesions, with a visible muscle blunt, with a "bell tongue" aspect (**Figure 14**).

On US examination, normal muscle is slightly hypoechogenic with hyperechoic septa and fascia [17]. In transverse plane, muscle tissue will normally have a "starry night appearance", while in long axis fibers run parallel to each other and at an angle towards the muscle insertion. Patients with inflammatory myopathies, such as polymyositis, dermatomyositis and inclusion body myositis, will display changes in muscle echogenicity. In acute phases, muscle edema will cause thickening and only slight increase in echogenicity which proves reversible to treatment [63]. In later

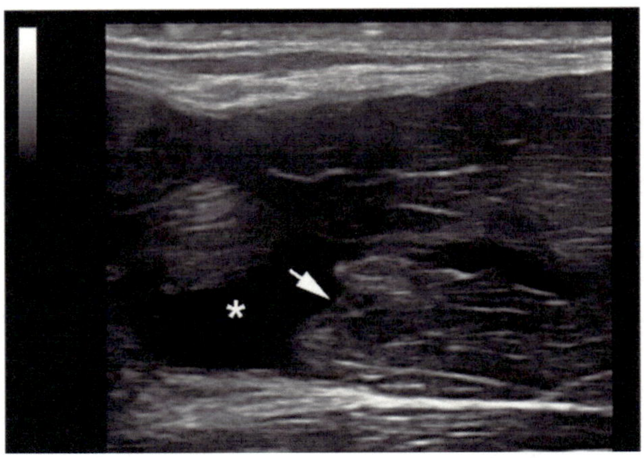

Figure 14.
Ultrasonography of the pectoralis major muscle with a lesion. Asterisk – Effusion secondary to the hemorrhage, arrow – The pectoralis muscle blunt ("bell tongue" aspect).

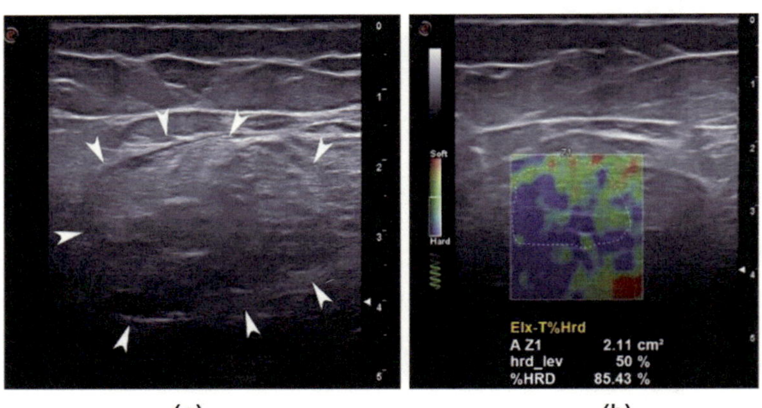

(a) (b)

Figure 15.
Ultrasonography of the rectus femoris in a patient with polymyositis, that shows increased echogenicity and lack of the starry night appearance in GS mode (a), and decreased elasticity as showed by the blue color in elastography and the hardness percent (b).

stages, ultrasound will detect markedly increased echogenicity, muscle atrophy and reduced elasticity (**Figure 15**).

Studies have observed correlations between US and histopathology and also significant changes in muscle stiffness when applying elastographic modalities. Patients with active myositis display increased stiffness and this will be gradually reduced as more severe muscle weakness develops [64].

Author details

Stefan Cristian Dinescu[1], Razvan Adrian Ionescu[2], Horatiu Valeriu Popoviciu[3], Claudiu Avram[4] and Florentin Ananu Vreju[1]*

1 Department of Rheumatology, University of Medicine and Pharmacy of Craiova, Romania

2 3d Internal Medicine Department, Carol Davila University of Medicine and Pharmacy Bucuresti, Romania

3 Department of Rheumatology, BFK and Medical Rehabilitation, University of Medicine, Pharmacy, Science and Technology of Targu Mures, Targu Mures, Romania

4 Department of Physical Therapy and Special Motricity, West University of Timisoara, Timisoara, Romania

*Address all correspondence to: florin_vreju@yahoo.com

References

[1] Colebatch AN, Edwards CJ, Østergaard M, van der Heijde D, Balint PV, D'Agostino MA, et al. EULAR recommendations for the use of imaging of the joints in the clinical management of rheumatoid arthritis. Annals of the Rheumatic Diseases. 2013;**72**(6):804-814. DOI: 10.1136/annrheumdis-2012-203158

[2] Mandl P, Navarro-Compán V, Terslev L, Aegerter P, van der Heijde D, D'Agostino MA, et al. EULAR recommendations for the use of imaging in the diagnosis and management of spondyloarthritis in clinical practice. Annals of the Rheumatic Diseases. 2015;**74**(7):1327-1339

[3] Möller I, Janta I, Backhaus M, Ohrndorf S, Bong David A, Martinoli C, et al. The 2017 EULAR standardised procedures for ultrasound imaging in rheumatology. Annals of the Rheumatic Diseases. 2017;**0**:1-6

[4] Wakefield RJ, Balint PV, Szkudlarek M, Filippucci E, Backhaus M, D'agostino M-A, et al. Musculoskeletal ultrasound including definitions for Ultrasonographic pathology. The Journal of Rheumatology. 2005;**32**(12):2485-2487

[5] Chen C, Cheng Y, Zhu X, Cai Y, Xue Y, Kong N, et al. Ultrasound assessment of skin thickness and stiffness: The correlation with histology and clinical score in systemic sclerosis. Arthritis Research & Therapy. 2020;**22**(1):197. DOI: 10.1186/s13075-020-02285-x

[6] Schmidt WA. Ultrasound in the diagnosis and management of giant cell arteritis. Rheumatology. 2018;**57**(suppl_2):ii22-ii31

[7] Jousse-Joulin S, Milic V, Jonsson MV, Plagou A, Theander E, Luciano N, et al. Is salivary gland ultrasonography a useful tool in Sjögren's syndrome? A systematic review. Rheumatology. 2016;**55**(5):789-800

[8] Vreju FA, Ciurea ME, Popa D, Popa F, Parvanescu CD, Chisalau BA, et al. Ultrasonography in the diagnosis and management of non inflammatory conditions of the hand and wrist. Medical Ultrasonography. 2016;**18**(1): 90-95

[9] Vreju F, Ciurea M, Roşu A, Muşetescu A, Grecu D, Ciurea P. Power Doppler sonography, a non-invasive method of assessment of the synovial inflammation in patients with early rheumatoid arthritis. Romanian Journal of Morphology and Embryology. 2011;**52**(2):637-643

[10] Zhao C-Y, Jiang Y-X, Li J-C, Xu Z-H, Zhang Q, Su N, et al. Role of contrast-enhanced ultrasound in the evaluation of inflammatory arthritis. Chinese Medical Journal. 2017;**130**(14):1722

[11] Bakewell CJ, Olivieri I, Aydin SZ, Dejaco C, Ikeda K, Gutierrez M, et al. Ultrasound and magnetic resonance imaging in the evaluation of psoriatic dactylitis: Status and perspectives. The Journal of Rheumatology. 2013;**40**(12): 1951-1957. DOI: 10.3899/jrheum.130643

[12] Sifuentes-Cantú C, Contreras-Yáñez I, Saldarriaga L, Lozada AC, Gutiérrez M, Pascual-Ramos V. The added value of musculoskeletal ultrasound to clinical evaluation in the treatment decision of rheumatoid arthritis outpatients: Physician experience matters. BMC Musculoskeletal Disorders. 2017;**18**(1): 1-10

[13] Klauser A, Halpern EJ, Frauscher F, Gvozdic D, Duftner C, Springer P, et al. Inflammatory low back pain: High negative predictive value of contrast-enhanced color Doppler ultrasound in the detection of inflamed sacroiliac

joints. Arthritis and Rheumatism. 2005;**53**(3):440-444. DOI: 10.1002/art.21161

[14] Klauser A, Demharter J, De Marchi A, Sureda D, Barile A, Masciocchi C, et al. Contrast enhanced gray-scale sonography in assessment of joint vascularity in rheumatoid arthritis: Results from the IACUS study group. European Radiology. 2005;**15**(12): 2404-2410

[15] Liu H, Huang C, Chen S, Zheng Q, Ye Y, Ye Z, et al. Value of contrast-enhanced ultrasound for detection of synovial vascularity in experimental rheumatoid arthritis: An exploratory study. The Journal of International Medical Research. 2019;**47**(11):5740-5751. DOI: 10.1177/0300060519874159

[16] Alfuraih AM, O'Connor P, Tan AL, Hensor EMA, Ladas A, Emery P, et al. Muscle shear wave elastography in idiopathic inflammatory myopathies: A case-control study with MRI correlation. Skeletal Radiology. 2019;**48**(8):1209-1219

[17] Kang T, Horton L, Emery P, Wakefield RJ. Value of ultrasound in rheumatologic diseases. Journal of Korean Medical Science. 2013;**28**: 497-507

[18] Ren J, Zhu J, Li D, Li W, Liu F. The value of contrast-enhanced ultrasonography to detect the sacroiliac joint for predicting relapse after discontinuation of anti-tumor necrosis factor therapy in patients with ankylosing spondylitis. Quantitative Imaging in Medicine and Surgery. 2019;**9**(6):1110

[19] Balea AM, Streba L, Vreju AF, Schenker M, Săndulescu DL, Bondari S, et al. Left gluteal metastasis from a hepatocellular carcinoma - an unusual finding. Romanian Journal of Morphology and Embryology. 2018;**59**(2):549-555

[20] Kane D, Grassi W, Sturrock R, Balint PV. Musculoskeletal ultrasound—A state of the art review in rheumatology. Part 2: Clinical indications for musculoskeletal ultrasound in rheumatology. Rheumatology. 2004;**43**(7):829-838

[21] Gutierrez M, Bertolazzi C, Castillo E, Reyes-Long S, Clavijo-Cornejo D, Santos-Moreno P. Ultrasound as a useful tool in the diagnosis of rheumatoid arthritis in patients with undifferentiated arthritis. Journal of Clinical Rheumatology. 2019;**25**(5):203-208

[22] Barbulescu AL, Ciurea PL, Mitran C, Chisalau BA, Parvanescu CD, Firulescu SC, et al. High frequency ultrasonography of the hand versus anti-RA33 evaluation in early rheumatoid arthritis - a pilot study. Medical Ultrasonography. 2017;**19**(2):166-171

[23] Di Matteo A, Mankia K, Azukizawa M, Wakefield RJ. The role of musculoskeletal ultrasound in the rheumatoid arthritis continuum. Current Rheumatology Reports. 2020;**22**(8):41. DOI: 10.1007/s11926-020-00911-w

[24] Iagnocco A, Ceccarelli F, Perricone C, Valesini G. The role of ultrasound in rheumatology. Seminars in Ultrasound, CT and MRI. 2011;**32**(2):66-73

[25] Lillegraven S, Bøyesen P, Hammer HB, Østergaard M, Uhlig T, Sesseng S, et al. Tenosynovitis of the extensor carpi ulnaris tendon predicts erosive progression in early rheumatoid arthritis. Annals of the Rheumatic Diseases. 2011;**70**(11):2049-2050

[26] Vreju FA, Filippucci E, Gutierrez M, di Geso L, Ciapetti A, Ciurea ME, et al. Subclinical ultrasound synovitis in a particular joint is associated with ultrasound evidence of bone erosions in that same joint in rheumatoid patients

in clinical remission. Clinical and Experimental Rheumatology. 2016;**34**:673-678

[27] Płaza M, Nowakowska-Płaza A, Pracoń G, Sudoł-Szopińska I. Role of ultrasonography in the diagnosis of rheumatic diseases in light of ACR/EULAR guidelines. Journal of Ultrasonography. 2016;**16**(64):55

[28] D'Agostino M-A, Terslev L, Aegerter P, Backhaus M, Balint P, Bruyn GA, et al. Original article: Scoring ultrasound synovitis in rheumatoid arthritis: A EULAR-OMERACT ultrasound taskforce—Part 1: Definition and development of a standardised, consensus-based scoring system. RMD Open. 2017;**3**(1):428

[29] Døhn UM, Terslev L, Szkudlarek M, Hansen MS, Hetland ML, Hansen A, et al. Detection, scoring and volume assessment of bone erosions by ultrasonography in rheumatoid arthritis: Comparison with CT. Annals of the Rheumatic Diseases. 2013;**72**(4): 530-534. DOI: 10.1136/annrheumdis-2011-201114

[30] Naredo E, D'Agostino MA, Wakefield RJ, Möller I, Balint PV, Filippucci E, et al. Reliability of a consensus-based ultrasound score for tenosynovitis in rheumatoid arthritis. Annals of the Rheumatic Diseases. 2013;**72**(8):1328-1334

[31] Backhaus M, Ohrndorf S, Kellner H, Strunk J, Backhaus TM, Hartung W, et al. Evaluation of a novel 7-joint ultrasound score in daily rheumatologic practice: A pilot project. Arthritis and Rheumatism. 2009;**61**(9):1194-1201. DOI: 10.1002/art.24646

[32] Damjanov N, Radunovic G, Prodanovic S, Vukovic V, Milic V, Simic Pasalic K, et al. Construct validity and reliability of ultrasound disease activity score in assessing joint inflammation in RA: Comparison with DAS-28. Rheumatology (Oxford, England). 2012;**51**(1):120-128. DOI: 10.1093/rheumatology/ker255

[33] Zabotti A, Salvin S, Quartuccio L, De Vita S. Differentiation between early rheumatoid and early psoriatic arthritis by the ultrasonographic study of the synovio-entheseal complex of the small joints of the hands. Clinical and Experimental Rheumatology. 2016;**34**(3):459-465

[34] Balint PV, Terslev L, Aegerter P, Bruyn GAW, Chary-Valckenaere I, Gandjbakhch F, et al. D'Agostino MA; OMERACT ultrasound task force members. Reliability of a consensus-based ultrasound definition and scoring for enthesitis in spondyloarthritis and psoriatic arthritis: An OMERACT US initiative. Annals of the Rheumatic Diseases. 2018;**77**(12):1730-1735. DOI: 10.1136/annrheumdis-2018-213609

[35] Gutierrez M, Filippucci E, De Angelis R, Filosa G, Kane D, Grassi W. A sonographic spectrum of psoriatic arthritis: "the five targets". Clinical Rheumatology. 2010;**29**(2):133-142. DOI: 10.1007/s10067-009-1292-y

[36] Kaeley GS. Enthesitis in psoriatic arthritis (part 2): Imaging. Rheumatology. 2020;**59** (Supplement_1):i15-i20

[37] Balint PV, Kane D, Wilson H, McInnes IB, Sturrock RD. Ultrasonography of entheseal insertions in the lower limb in spondyloarthropathy. Annals of the Rheumatic Diseases. 2002;**61**(10): 905-910. DOI: 10.1136/ard.61.10.905

[38] Macía-Villa C, Falcao S, Medina J, De Miguel E. Ultrasonography of enthesis in psoriatic arthritis: A descriptive and reliability analysis of elemental lesions and power Doppler subtypes. Scandinavian Journal of Rheumatology. 2019;**48**(6):454-459. DOI: 10.1080/03009742.2019.1602881

[39] Tom S, Zhong Y, Cook R, Aydin SZ, Kaeley G, Eder L. Development of a preliminary Ultrasonographic Enthesitis score in psoriatic arthritis - GRAPPA ultrasound working group. The Journal of Rheumatology. 2019;**46**(4):384-390. DOI: 10.3899/jrheum.171465

[40] Benjamin M, McGonagle D. The anatomical basis for disease localisation in seronegative spondyloarthropathy at entheses and related sites. Journal of Anatomy. 2001;**199**(Pt 5):503-526

[41] Zabotti A, Sakellariou G. Tinazzi I, et alNovel and reliable DACTylitis glObal sonographic (DACTOS) score in psoriatic arthritis. Annals of the Rheumatic Diseases. 2020;**79**:1037-1043

[42] Girolimetto N, Giovannini I, Crepaldi G, De MG, Tinazzi I, Possemato N, et al. Psoriatic Dactylitis: Current perspectives and new insights in ultrasonography and magnetic resonance imaging. Journal of Clinical Medicine. 2021;**10**(12):2604

[43] Girolimetto N, Zabotti A, Tinazzi I, Possemato N, Costa L, Batticciotto A, et al. Sensitivity to change and clinical correlations of the novel DACtylitis glObal sonographic (DACTOS) score in psoriatic arthritis. Rheumatology. 2021;**60**(9):4103-4111

[44] Grassi W, Meenagh G, Pascual E, Filippucci E. "Crystal clear"- sonographic assessment of gout and calcium pyrophosphate deposition disease. Seminars in Arthritis and Rheumatism. 2006;**36**:197-202

[45] Christiansen SN, Østergaard M, Terslev L. Ultrasonography in gout: Utility in diagnosis and monitoring. Clinical and Experimental Rheumatology. 2018;**36**:S61-S67

[46] Neogi T, Jansen TLTA, Dalbeth N, Fransen J, Schumacher HR, Berendsen D, et al. 2015 gout classification criteria: An American College of Rheumatology/European league against rheumatism collaborative initiative. Annals of the Rheumatic Diseases. 2015;**74**(10):1789-1798

[47] Zhang W, Doherty M, Bardin T, Barskova V, Guerne PA, Jansen TL, et al. European league against rheumatism recommendations for calcium pyrophosphate deposition. Part I: Terminology and diagnosis. Annals of the Rheumatic Diseases. 2011;**70**(4):563-570. DOI: 10.1136/ard.2010.139105

[48] Filippou G, Scanu A, Adinolfi A, Toscano C, Gambera D, Largo R, et al. Criterion validity of ultrasound in the identification of calcium pyrophosphate crystal deposits at the knee: An OMERACT ultrasound study. Annals of the Rheumatic Diseases. 2020;**80**(2): 261-267

[49] Filippou G, Scirè CA, Damjanov N, Adinolfi A, Carrara G, Picerno V, et al. Definition and reliability assessment of elementary ultrasonographic findings in calcium pyrophosphate deposition disease: A study by the OMERACT calcium pyrophosphate deposition disease ultrasound subtask force. The Journal of Rheumatology. 2017;**44**(11): 1744-1749

[50] Filippou G, Scirè CA, Adinolfi A, Damjanov NS, Carrara G, Bruyn GAW, et al. Identification of calcium pyrophosphate deposition disease (CPPD) by ultrasound: Reliability of the OMERACT definitions in an extended set of joints - an international multiobserver study by the OMERACT calcium pyrophosphate deposition disease ultrasound. Annals of the Rheumatic Diseases. 2018;**77**(8):1195-1200

[51] Amorese-O'Connell L, Gutierrez M, Reginato AM. General applications of ultrasound in rheumatology practice. Federal Practitioner. 2015; **32**(Suppl. 12):8S

[52] Mortada M, Zeid A, Al-Toukhy MAE-H, Ezzeldin N, Elgawish M.

Reliability of a proposed Ultrasonographic grading scale for severity of primary knee osteoarthritis. Clinical Medicine Insights: Arthritis and Musculoskeletal Disorders. 2016;**9**:161-166

[53] Moore TL, Lunt M, McManus B, Anderson ME, Herrick AL. Seventeen-point dermal ultrasound scoring system—A reliable measure of skin thickness in patients with systemic sclerosis. Rheumatology. 2003;**42**(12): 1559-1563

[54] Li H, Furst DE, Jin H, Sun C, Wang X, Yang L, et al. High-frequency ultrasound of the skin in systemic sclerosis: An exploratory study to examine correlation with disease activity and to define the minimally detectable difference. Arthritis Research & Therapy. 2018;**20**(1):1-8

[55] Yang Y, Qiu L, Wang L, Xiang X, Tang Y, Li H, et al. Quantitative assessment of skin stiffness using ultrasound shear wave Elastography in systemic sclerosis. Ultrasound in Medicine & Biology. 2019;**45**(4): 902-912. DOI: 10.1016/j.ultrasmedbio. 2018.11.015

[56] Carotti M, Salaffi F, Di Carlo M, Barile A, Giovagnoni A. Diagnostic value of major salivary gland ultrasonography in primary Sjögren's syndrome: The role of grey-scale and colour/power Doppler sonography. Gland Surgery. 2019;**8**(Suppl. 3):S159

[57] Lee KA, Lee SH, Kim HR. Diagnostic and predictive evaluation using salivary gland ultrasonography in primary Sjögren's syndrome. Clinical and Experimental Rheumatology. 2018;**36**:S165-S172

[58] De Vita S, Lorenzon G, Rossi G, Sabella M, Fossaluzza V. Salivary gland echography in primary and secondary Sjögren's syndrome. Clinical and Experimental Rheumatology. 1992;**10**(4):351-356

[59] Hočevar A, Ambrožič A, Rozman B, Kveder T, Tomšič M. Ultrasonographic changes of major salivary glands in primary Sjögren's syndrome. Diagnostic value of a novel scoring system. Rheumatology. 2005;**44**(6):768-772

[60] Salaffi F, Carotti M, Iagnocco A, Luccioli F, Ramonda R, Sabatini E, et al. Ultrasonography of salivary glands in primary Sjögren's syndrome: A comparison with contrast sialography and scintigraphy. Rheumatology (Oxford, England). 2008;**47**(8): 1244-1249

[61] El Miedany YM, Ahmed I, Mourad HG, Mehanna AN, Aty SA, Gamal HM, et al. Quantitative ultrasonography and magnetic resonance imaging of the parotid gland: Can they replace the histopathologic studies in patients with Sjogren's syndrome? Joint Bone Spine. 2004;**71**(1):29-38

[62] Hellmich B, Agueda A, Monti S, Buttgereit F, De Boysson H, Brouwer E, et al. 2018 update of the EULAR recommendations for the management of large vessel vasculitis. Annals of the Rheumatic Diseases. 2020;**79**(1):19-30

[63] Albayda J, van Alfen N. Diagnostic value of muscle ultrasound for myopathies and myositis. Current Rheumatology Reports. 2020;**22**(11):82

[64] Botar-Jid C, Damian L, Dudea SM, Vasilescu D, Rednic S, Badea R. The contribution of ultrasonography and sonoelastography in assessment of myositis. Medical Ultrasonography. 2010;**12**(2):120-126

Chapter 6

Value of Breast Ultrasound in the Clinical Practice of the Surgeon

María Eugenia Aponte-Rueda and María Isabel de Abreu

Abstract

In recent years, breast surgeons have been increasing the use of ultrasound as a reliable and useful tool in their practice to assist in managing patients and the operating room. An appropriate clinical and sonographic correlation can define diagnostic workup, provide immediate reassurance to the patients, and perform one-site diagnostic needle interventions. Particularly, it has a significant role in low-middle income countries, where imaging services are scarce due to its high cost, maintenance needs, and limited availability of trained personnel. Therefore, training and accreditation of surgeons who perform and interpret ultrasound are required interventions to influence the provider's knowledge, accomplish optimal practices, complete diagnostic examinations of the breast, and improve the patients' quality of care. This review aims to serve as an educational resource regarding the up-to-date value of breast ultrasound for surgeons.

Keywords: Breast Ultrasound, Breast Imaging, Interventional Radiology, Breast Cancer, Intraoperative Ultrasound, Low and Middle Income Countries, Breast Surgeon

1. Introduction

Ultrasound (US) is a reliable and helpful tool in evaluating, diagnosing, and managing breast disease improving the patients' quality of care. In recent years, with the increasing quality of the ultrasonography equipment, the surgeons have escalated its use, particularly by breast surgeons in their clinical practice and operating room, which has led to the enhanced provision of care for women with breast disease [1, 2].

Breast ultrasound allows immediate identification and characterization of localized breast symptoms, palpable abnormalities noted on physical breast examination; and nonpalpable abnormalities identified on other breast imaging modalities. Hence, an appropriate clinical and sonographic correlation can define diagnostic workup, provide immediate reassurance to the patients, and perform one-site diagnostic needle interventions. In addition, it has the advantages of being low-cost, more affordable, portable, safe, and requires minimal maintenance. It has a significant role in low-middle income countries, where imaging services are scarce due to its high cost and limited availability of trained personnel [3]. In these settings, capacities on local referral chains are minimal; therefore, the use of US by breast surgeons offers significant appropriateness to the patients by allowing them to obviate the high threshold needed to reach referral services.

Breast surgeons can acquire comprehensive skills and competence in US techniques and their indications in the outpatient setting under the supervision of a

US-experienced radiologist or surgeon, enhancing the multidisciplinary care of breast patients. Also, participation in training courses guided by local proficiency standards [1] allows the successful incorporation of breast ultrasound and ultrasound-guided breast procedures into clinical practice, which can then be translated into the operation room. Training and accreditation of surgeons who perform and interpret ultrasound is an intervention that influences providers' behavior for optimal patient outcomes. Hence, the surgeon who assists in managing breast patients has to design a rational plan of action based on their knowledge, available resources, and patient needs to ensure adequate and safe breast care [4–6].

The purpose of this review is to serve as an educational resource for the value of breast ultrasound in the clinical practice of the surgeon by providing the understanding of its applications for the evaluation, management, and monitoring of breast diseases; and the recognizing of its indications for interventional breast procedures in order to improve the decision-making process and enhance patient care.

2. Indications of breast ultrasound

Breast ultrasound is valuable in several clinical situations, including but not limited to the following [4, 5, 7]:

- Identification and characterization of localized breast symptoms, palpable abnormalities noted on clinical breast examination, and nonpalpable abnormalities identified on other breast imaging modalities.

- Initial Imaging evaluation of localized breast symptoms and palpable abnormalities in patients under 40 years of age who are not at risk of developing breast cancer and in lactating or pregnant women.

- Evaluation and characterization of abnormalities associated with breast implants.

- Guidance for breast interventional or surgical procedures.

- Preoperative evaluation of the breast and axilla in diagnosed breast cancer.

- Evaluation and assessment of the breast after surgical or medical therapy.

- Intraoperative ultrasound-guided breast surgery and intraoperative assessment of lumpectomy margins.

3. Breast ultrasound overview

Breast Ultrasound is a diagnostic tool that makes the whole imaging assessment more specific and expedited. Alongside clinical information, US characterization allows imaging correlation to define further imaging workup and recommend interventional procedures for diagnostic and therapeutic purposes. Ultrasound is called hand-held or manual when the probe is manually moved on the breast surface (HHUS). In automated whole breast ultrasonography (ABUS), the probe scans the whole breast in a standard fashion, gathering and storing a set of images for later review by physicians interpreting the findings [8].

DOI: http://dx.doi.org/10.5772/intechopen.100520

3.1 Reporting system

The Breast Imaging Reporting and Data System® (BI-RADS®) is a management system developed for imaging that contains: (1) a lexicon of descriptors, i.e., a dictionary of specific imaging features; (2) a standardized reporting structure-including final assessment categories with accompanying recommendations; (3) a framework for data collection and auditing. This system aids communication and comprehension of imaging findings by all members of the multidisciplinary breast care team: surgeons, pathologists, oncologists, radiologists, and other health care providers. BI-RADS final assessment categories and their recommendations have become the standard by which physicians determine breast care, allowing uniform drafting of reports, facilitating the research, and performance evaluation [9].

These categories, currently are as follows [10]:

- Category 0: Incomplete. Need additional imaging evaluation or previous images for comparison to determine appropriate management and final assessment.

- Category 1: Negative. There is no US imaging abnormality. Routine screening.

- Category 2: Benign Findings. Negative for malignancy. No further investigation is required based on the imaging finding. Routine screening.

- Category 3: Indeterminate/Probably Benign Finding. Lesions with less than 2% risk of malignancy. Should recommend initial short-interval follow-up.

- Category 4: Suspicious Abnormality. Lesions with >2% but <95% likelihood of malignancy. Diagnostic tissue sampling through biopsy should be performed in the absence of clinical contraindication— 4A (low suspicion for malignancy, >2% but ≤10% likelihood of malignancy), 4B (moderate suspicion for malignancy, >10% but ≥50% likelihood of malignancy), and 4C (high suspicion for malignancy, >50% but <95% likelihood of malignancy).

- Category 5: US findings highly suggestive of malignancy. More than 95% likelihood of malignancy. Diagnostic tissue sampling through biopsy should be performed in the absence of clinical contraindication.

- Category 6: Known biopsy-proven malignancy. Reserved for US examinations performed for cancer staging or monitoring of neoadjuvant therapy.

Similarly, in the UK, the Royal College of Radiologists Breast Group (RCRBG) [11] has developed a five-point scoring system to classify breast images, using a similar rationale to the American College of Radiologists' development of the BI-RADS®. However, this classification does not specify the probable cancer risk of each category. This five-point system is Normal (category 1)- there are no significant imaging findings. Benign findings (category 2)- the benign imaging findings are not indicated for further investigation. Indeterminate / probably benign (category 3)- low risk of malignancy, and further investigation through needle biopsy is indicated. Findings suspicious of malignancy (category 4)- show a moderate risk of malignancy, so further investigation is indicated through a needle biopsy. Highly suspicious findings of malignancy (category 5)- high risk of malignancy; further investigation is indicated through a needle biopsy.

3.2 Imaging quality

The US is a highly operator-dependent technique due to a lack of repetitiveness and a strong reliance on specialists' abilities and judgment to capture the right image to be documented in the report. Although the ACRIN 6666 trial has proposed a model, no standard US acquisition technique exists yet [12]. A specialist with competence and experience should perform breast ultrasound [13, 14], correlating clinical signs or symptoms, mammographic studies, and other breast imaging. If the ultrasound has been performed previously, the current examination should be compared with a previous ultrasound, as appropriate.

3.3 Setting

The correct application of the vocabulary depends on the quality of the ultrasound equipment, ultrasound technique, and an adequate compression of the breast anatomy. Breast ultrasound should be performed with high-resolution linear array transducers from 7.5–8 (at least) to 15–18 MHz. Higher frequency is recommended for less depth penetration (superficial details or small breasts). Lower frequency should be used for deeper areas or very large breasts (4 to 8 MHz) [5]. An acoustic stand-off pad is useful for superficial images. It is critical to document and capture appropriate imaging for actionable cases by optimizing focal zone selections, gain settings, and view fields. When a potential finding is located, turn the transducer to assess if it persists and better characterize it. A wide-band linear matrix transducer offers better resolution by focusing on the short axis.

3.4 Positioning

The patient should be lying in the supine position placed with the chest undressed. There are two breast survey patient positions: a medial position with the ipsilateral arm overhead or with arms flexed behind the head to flatten the breast, and an oblique position with a wedge supporting the back for scanning the lateral part of the breast and the axilla. Scan techniques should allow systematic exploration of the entire breast, whether grid scanning or radial scanning patterns.

3.5 Labeling

Images should be labeled as right or left breast and should be reported the transducer orientation. The localization of the findings is described by quadrant -upper external, lower external, lower internal, upper internal- and retroareolar region; or according to the clock-wise position (distance from the nipple). Distance from the nipple to the lesion should not be measured from the areola's edge since the areolar width is variable [5]. A large lesion can be captured in a single image by Panoramic Imaging (Extended Field of View –FOV-) and traced the lesion back to the nipple for an accurate distance reporting.

3.6 Measurements

All lesions are measured in three dimensions, including length, width, and height unless shadowing disguises the accurate height measurement. Dimensions must register with the greatest millimeter or centimeter accuracy. The first measurement represents the longest axis. The following measurement is perpendicular to the long axis, and the last measurement is from an orthogonal projection to the first image (representing a different plane from the former two images). It is necessary to capture two sets of lesion images (one with calipers and one without) [6, 10].

Solid masses diagnosed as benign pathology may safely have periodic surveillance if the volume growth rate is less than 16% per month in women under 50 years and less than 13% per month in women 50 years or older. An acceptable mean change for three dimensions during a six-month interval is 20% for all ages [15].

3.7 Documentation

Accurate documentation is essential for high-quality patient care. Ultrasound report is only as good as the images on which it is based. Images and reports are part of the patient's medical record. Each image should have the facility name, date of examination, patient's first and last name, identification number, and birth date. It should display identification of left or right breast and lesion's location. It should indicate transducer orientation within the breast (radial, antiradial, oblique, transversal, or sagittal), distance from the nipple, and three orthogonal measurements. Breast ultrasound document must contain the following sections [5, 6, 10]:

- Indication of breast ultrasound.
- Description of the scope and technique of breast ultrasound.
- Brief description of the overall composition of the breasts.
- A detailed description of important findings.
- Comparison with prior relevant imaging studies and correlation with signs observed during the clinical examination.
- Assessment and management recommendations.
- Report of ultrasound-guided interventional procedures should include the location of the lesion, the approach, the type of prep and local anesthesia, the skin incision, the type of device used, the number of cores taken, and the type of clip placed, if any. Whenever specimen radiographs or sonograms are performed, they should be recorded in the report.

4. Breast ultrasound lexicon

Descriptors for breast tissue composition (background echotexture) are correlated to mammographic breast densities. These are homogeneous-fat, homogenous-fibroglandular, and heterogeneous. In Homogeneous-fat background, fat lobules and echogenic bands of supporting structures comprise the bulk of the breast tissue. In the Homogeneous-fibroglandular background, a dense zone of the homogeneously echogenic bands of fibroglandular parenchyma is present beneath the thin hypoechogenic layer of fat lobules. Heterogeneous background echotexture is characterized by multiple small areas of increased or decreased echogenicity, either focal or diffuse.

For the identification and characterization of the masses, the number of characteristics to be described are seven: *shape* (oval, round, and irregular), *orientation* (parallel and not parallel), *margins* (circumscribed and not circumscribed, indistinct, angular, microlobulated, and spiculated), *echo pattern* (anechoic, hyperechoic, complex cystic and solid, hypoechoic, isoechoic and heterogeneous) *posterior acoustic features* (no posterior acoustic features, enhancement, shadowing and combined pattern), *calcifications* (in or outside of a mass, and intraductal) and *associated features*.

Associated features include architectural distortion; edema; duct changes; skin changes (skin retraction, skin thickening-focal and diffuse-); vascularity (absent, internal, and vessel in rim), and elasticity assessment. Elasticity assessment of tissue stiffness (elastography) explores modifications of the US image of a lesion after applying a manual compression (strain) or introducing ultrasonic energy (shear wave). Applicable descriptors are color-codes tissue hardness. The elasticity assessment is a feature available on many modern US units and included in the last BI-RADS edition. The World Federation of Ultrasound in Medicine and Biology (WFUMB) has published guidelines in characterizing breast lesions as benign or malignant, although this fact cannot be misinterpreted as an entire endorsement of the clinical validity of elasticity assessment. Therefore, the elastography should be integrated for patient management alongside the more predictive ultrasonic morphologic features of malignancy (shape, margin, and echogenicity). Currently, the share-wave elastography is used as a valuable preoperative predictor of chemotherapy response [16].

It is essential to analyze several features, rather than just one, for lesion categorization as benign or malignant. Benign and malignant solid masses can equally be well-differentiated on ultrasound. Benign US features include an oval shape, well-circumscribed margins, and parallel orientation to the skin. Suspicious US features include irregular margins, marked hypoechogenicity, post-acoustic shadowing, and non-parallel orientation to the skin (**Figure 1**).

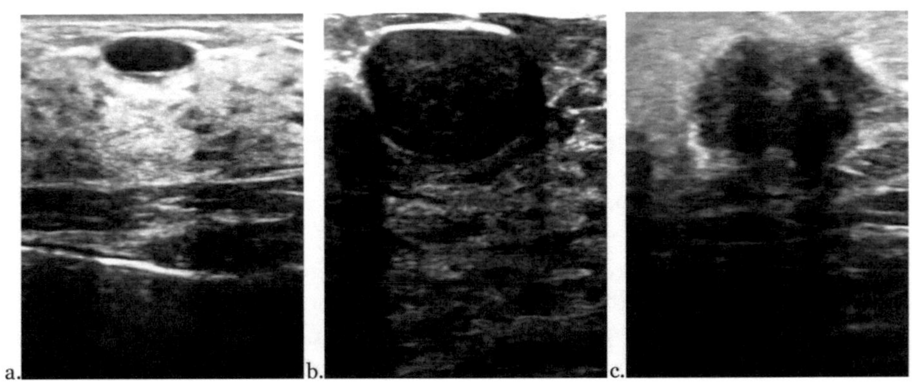

Figure 1.
Ultrasound characteristics of breast lesions. (a) Circumscribed, oval, anechoic mass with parallel orientation and posterior enhancement consistent with a simple cyst. (b) Circumscribed, round, heterogeneous mass with lateral shadowing. The pathological diagnosis by biopsy was Fibroadenoma. (c) Irregular, noncircumscribed, hypoechoic mass with posterior shadowing: Invasive Breast Carcinoma by biopsy.

5. Identification and characterization of palpable breast symptoms

5.1 Nipple discharge

Clinical workup of nipple discharge includes a detailed patient medical history, recently recorded trauma, careful physical examination, and the most suitable breast imaging modality. The evaluation and management aim of nipple discharge is to identify the causative condition accurately, distinguishing between "pathologic" causes from those with "benign or physiological" causes, and consequently diagnosing cancer when it is present.

The discharge's clinical characteristics should describe color, whether uni or bilateral or associated with nipple stimulation or breast compression, whether it originated from a single duct or multiple ducts [17]. Benign nipple discharge is traditionally considered bilateral, non-spontaneous, emanating from multiple ducts after manipulation or stimulation; varies in color from white to yellow to green to brown. Pathologic discharge is considered unilateral, spontaneous, persistent, clear, serous, serosanguinous, or bloody from a single duct [18].

Breast imaging identifies and characterizes any lesion in these patients and assists subsequent percutaneous biopsy in achieving a histopathologic diagnosis [19]. Magnetic resonance imaging (MRI) may be useful in pathologic nipple discharge when lesions cannot be localized with other diagnostic imaging [20]. However, MRI is limited, and it is not yet a generalized practice because it is expensive and not readily available in all areas [21].

In patients with nipple discharge, the sensitivity of mammography in detecting an abnormality is low. The ability of mammograms to identify intraductal lesions is limited since they are generally small and lack microcalcifications. In mammography subareolar region usually shows increased density. The sensitivity and specificity of ultrasound vary from 36 to 83% and 12–84%, respectively. Several factors can explain this wide range, including differences in the criteria used to distinguish between pathologic from benign discharge and differences in ultrasound technology employed [22]. Breast US is useful for visualizing ductal structures, localization of the lesions that cause the nipple discharge, and the subsequent accomplishment of imaging-guided percutaneous biopsy to determine whether a malignant lesion is the cause of the pathologic nipple discharge. US-guided core needle biopsy in patients with pathologic nipple discharge, who had negative findings on mammography but had positive findings on US have reported 15.1% of cancer detection [23].

Breast US is capable of visualizing ductal structures located in the subareolar region. The BI-RADS® categorizes ductal changes as *associated features*. Duct changes are manifested by:

- cystic dilatation of a duct or ducts comprising irregular calibers or arborization. Dilated retroareolar duct is defined as duct ectasia, i.e., a duct with a diameter over 3 mm;
- extension of ducts to or from a malignant lesion; or
- intraductal mass, thrombus, or debris. Intraductal masses are assessed as category 4a, pointing out a requirement for biopsy because these have a risk of malignancy that cannot eliminate (**Figure 2**) [10, 24].

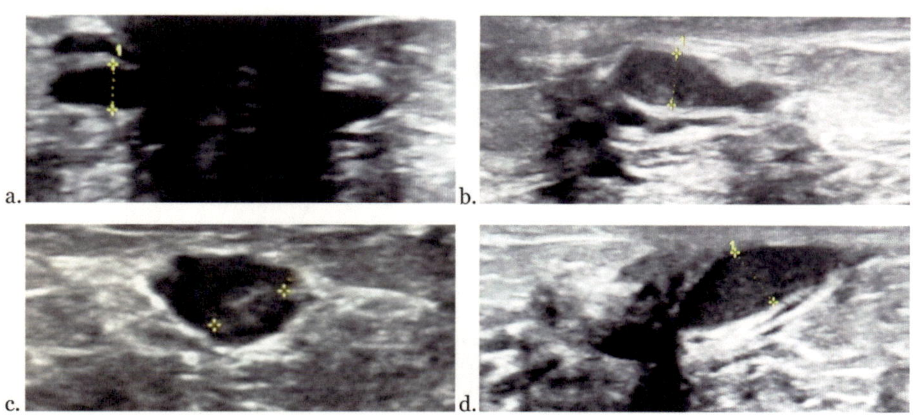

Figure 2.
(a) Single galactophere duct ectasia without any filling defect (calipers); (b) 49-year-old female with uniorificial serous nipple discharge. US: duct ectasia with echogenic content filled with thick secretion; (c) 46-year-old female with uniorificial bloody nipple discharge. US: single dilated duct with isoechoic endoductal mass with an ill-defined outline representing an intraductal papilloma by pathology report; (d) 39-year-old female with right uniorifical serosanguineous discharge. US: irregular intraductal mass arising from a dilated duct due to carcinoma in situ.

At present, there are no clear guidelines on which radiographic or clinical variables in patients with nipple discharge can predict malignancy. The malignancy rate in patients with nipple discharge ranges from 9.3–23% [18, 25–29]. However, these data were derived from studies made before improvements in breast ultrasound and the imaging-guided percutaneous biopsy. Most studies included patients referred to surgery departments or specialty breast centers [18, 25–27] or only those who underwent duct excision [28, 29].

Currently, less invasive diagnostic procedures affect the decision-making process about surgical management. For patients with pathological discharge and negative imaging evaluation (negative mammography results and negative features on breast US), surgical treatment has traditionally been indicated to eliminate symptoms and rule out breast carcinoma [24–28]. Although based on the low risk of underlying carcinoma, several studies have proposed conservative clinical follow-up and have shown that short-term monitoring would appear to be a reasonable approach in these patients [30, 31] Sabel et al. [31] suggested short-term observation with repeat imaging and clinical exam for low-risk patients (those without a strong family history or personal history of cancer). Ashfaq et al. [30] proposed a close clinical follow-up comprising a physical examination and breast ultrasound every six months for 1 to 2 years, or until the discharge resolved, whichever came first, plus annual mammography according to the screening guidelines. Patients who refuse to watch and wait as a clinical approach or report discomfort by the symptom or discharge after two years should consider the surgical treatment (**Figure 3**).

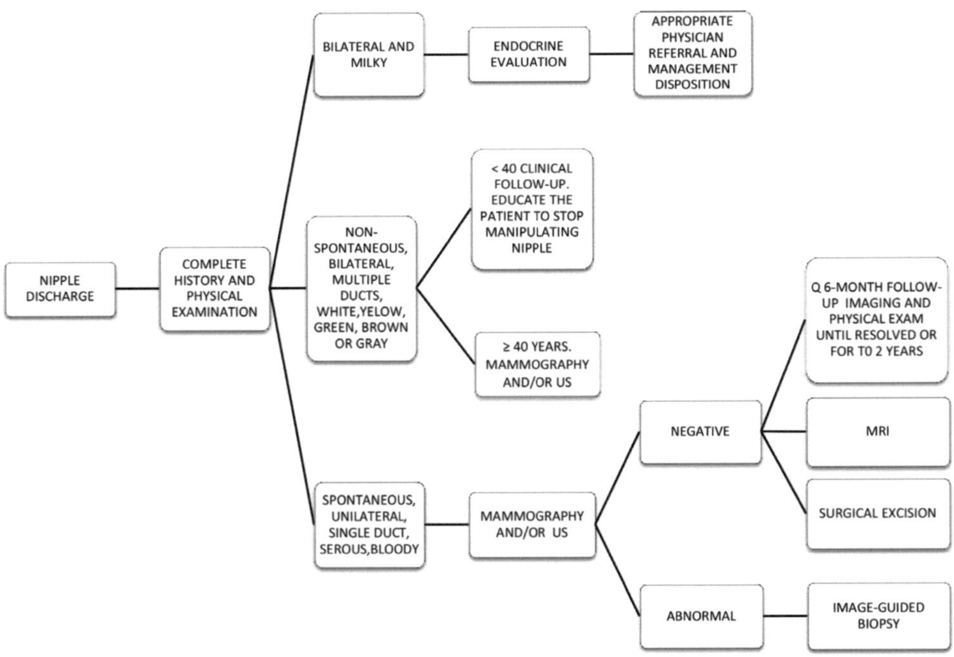

Figure 3.
Workflow for the management of women presenting with nipple discharge.

5.2 Inflammatory breast disease

Ultrasound examination is essential in evaluating patients with breast inflammation to identify fluid collections in the affected area by the inflammatory process and distinguish between cancer-related and non-cancer-related breast inflammation (since their clinical presentation can be misleading). Inflammatory breast disease manifests clinically by the cardinal signs of inflammation: redness, heat, and pain. It is classified as an infectious origin (generally bacterial) or non-infectious origin.

Breast US cardinal signs of infectious inflammatory breast disease are [32]:

- Skin thickening.
- Reticulated network of irregular hypoechoic lines, located at the interface between the dermis and subcutaneous fat, representing either dilated lymphatics or interstitial fluid.
- Increased echogenicity of surrounding fat tissue. Hyperechoic area extension is variable and depends on the degree of inflammation.
- Subcutaneous dilated vessels. Doppler signal demonstrates increased vascularity associated with hyperemia.
- Reactive lymphadenopathy: Enlarged axillary lymph nodes, regular cortical thickening, smooth borders, and visible central hilum.
- Ductal ectasia with thickened walls and echoic content into the duct (Galactophoritis).
- Breast abscess presents as round, oval or irregular; generally hypoechoic with multiples internal echoes, sometimes with fluid-debris level; usually with posterior acoustic enhancement. The walls may appear thickened with indistinct margins to the surrounding hyperechoic fat. An evident hypoechoic sinus tract probably extends the skin surface (Zuska's disease) [33]. It is a rare disease characterized by repeated and recurrent episodes of inflammatory abscesses and fistulae that is usually open on the edge of the areola or in the breast tissue close to it.

Ultrasound can be used to guide percutaneous sampling procedures and complete drainage of the fluid collection. If the collection is large (sizes >3 cm)- or if it remains or recurs-placing a percutaneous drainage catheter guided by US is the optimal course of the management [34]. In the unusual event of inadequate percutaneous drainage, surgical drainage should be an option.

Non-infectious inflammatory breast disease includes Granulomatous Mastitis and Diabetic Mastopathy. Diabetic Mastopathy appears as a hypoechoic mass with ill-defined margins and marked posterior shadowing.

Granulomatous Mastitis is a diagnosis of exclusion, and it is hardly made based on clinical signs and imaging findings. Clinical presentation is a firm to hard mass localized or diffused involvement of the entire breast with skin thickening, erythema, and inflammation (peau d' orange) that can clinically mimic carcinoma. In addition, the presence of draining sinus tracts and regional adenopathy are frequent. The diagnosis is established by histological analysis showing a granulomatous inflammatory response containing multinucleated giant cell granuloma. It is mainly seen in developing countries [35, 36]. Breast US signs in granulomatous mastitis are:

- Skin thickening

- Heterogeneously hypoechoic mass with poorly defined borders, with internal tubular hypoechoic structures.

- Parenchymal heterogeneity and architectural distortion with or without acoustic shadowing in the absence of a definite mass. Increased surrounding parenchymal vascularity on Doppler ultrasound.

- Enlarged axillary lymph nodes with reactive cortical thickening.

- Fluid collections with low-level internal echoes and hypoechoic sinus tracts extending to the skin in advanced cases (**Figure 4**).

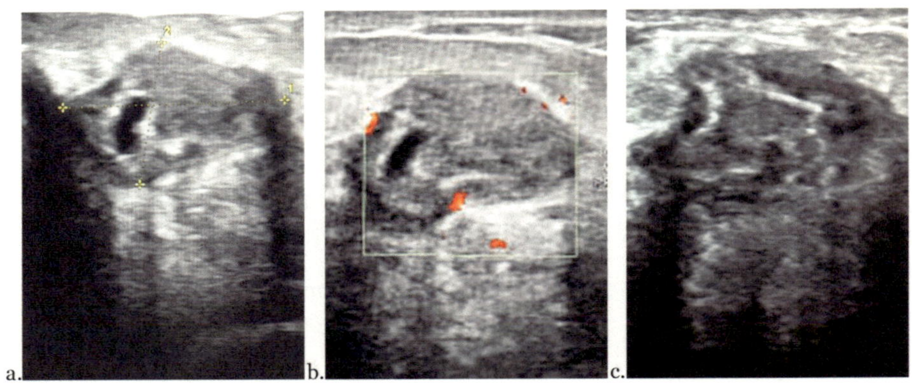

Figure 4.
45-year-old female with redness, heat, and pain in the right breast. US: (a) Hypoechoic mass with heterogeneous content, poorly defined borders, and acoustic shadowing. Thickening of the dermal layer. Fat hyperechogenicity around the mass. (b) Image using Doppler signal reveals increased surrounding vascularization. (c) US-Guided Percutaneous Biopsy: Granulomatous Mastitis.

5.3 Mass in breast skin

Lesions in the breast skin that arise within the dermal layer are considered generally benign. Most dermal lesions are palpable, providing the reason for imaging evaluations. Although occasionally, they are detected at screening imaging. This lesion includes dermal cysts, specifically sebaceous cysts and epidermal inclusion cysts (after a mammoplasty), for which routine surveillance is recommended..

Ultrasound findings of dermal lesions are [37]:

- An echogenic dermal layer surrounds lesions.

- A tract-to-skin from the lesion represents an extension of the hair follicle from the dermis through the epidermis.

- An acute or right angle (90 degrees) with the dermal line. A claw of hyper-echoic tissue wraps around the lesion's margin.

- Round well-circumscribed nodule or non-circumscribed-when inflammation is present-depending on its contents. The internal echotexture varies from anechoic to hypoechoic and heterogeneous (**Figure 5**).

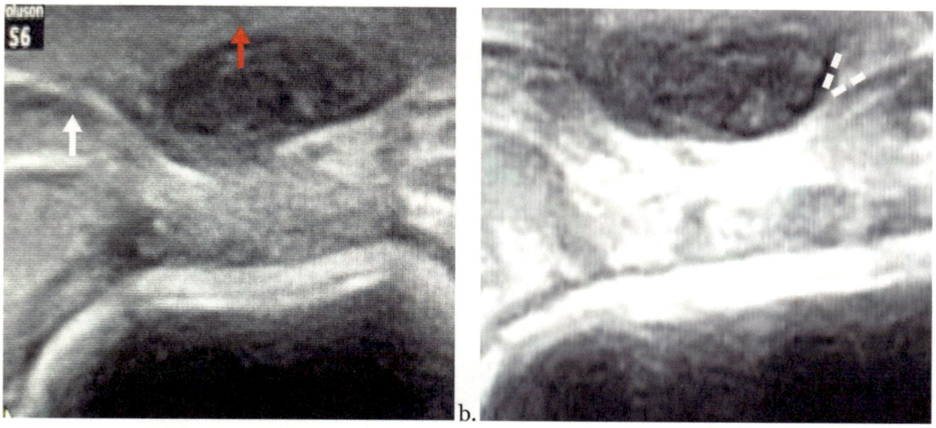

Figure 5.
57-year-old female with epidermal inclusion cyst located on the breast skin after mammoplasty. US: (a) hypoechoic well-circumscribed mass contained within the dermis. The dermal layer is thickened (white arrow) and extended into the hypodermis. A tract extends to the epidermal skin surface (red arrow). (b) The claw sign (white dashed line): dermal tissue wrapping around the margin of the lesion forming an acute angle.

6. Evaluation and characterization of abnormals associated with implants

In addition to the clinical examination, ultrasound is a useful diagnostic test to examine breast implant alterations, mainly ruptures. The breast implant is anechoic with an echogenic shell of a three-layered appearance (an anechogenic line between two echogenic lines). Small radial folds and a small amount of periprosthetic fluid are considered normal findings. US is very specific in evaluating breast implant integrity, albeit not very sensitive. The probability of rupture is highly suspected in US, but a rupture is still possible, even if it cannot be visible in US [7].

Alterations of the implant structure, classically, are *capsular contracture* or *capsular fibrosis* and *ruptures*. Capsular contracture is the capsule developed around the implant as the body's overreaction to a foreign device, leading to the hardening and deformation of the implant. There are three typical findings for capsular contracture or fibrosis: (1) *deformity*, not well evaluable with ultrasound (due to the narrow field of view), (2) *increased number of radial folds,* creating an undulated implant surface; and (3) *thickening of the fibrous capsule*, an echogenic line superficial to the implant shell, separated only by an anechoic line [38].

Ruptures are subdivided into intracapsular (implant envelope is broken, but containment remains inside the capsule) and extracapsular (when containment leaks out of the broken capsule) type [39]. The classic finding of extracapsular rupture of silicone implant on US is the snowstorm appearance, i.e., a highly echogenic pattern of scattered and reverberating echoes with a well-defined anterior margin. This appearance can also see in the axillary nodes containing free silicone. Intracapsular silicone implant rupture finding is the stepladder sign, characterized as a sequence of horizontal echogenic straight or curvilinear lines inside the collapsed implant shell [40]. If the prosthesis is saline, the collapsed implant shell will be evident by ultrasound.

According to the American College of Radiologists [41], breast implants evaluation varies on patient age, implant type, and symptoms. For patients less than 30 years with rupture of saline implants, ultrasound is the imaging choice. Mammography or US may be used for patients from 30 to 39 years of age with rupture of saline implants, and mammography is preferred for those 40 years and older. MRI without contrast or US is preferred for patients less than 30 years with rupture of silicone implants. MRI without contrast, mammography, or US may be used for those 30 to 39 years of age, and for those 40 years and older, MRI without contrast or mammography is used. Patients with unexplained axillary lymphadenopathy and silicone implants (current or previous) are assessed with the axillary US. Patients with suspected breast implant-associated anaplastic large-cell lymphoma should be recommended breast US, regardless of age or implant type.

7. Guidance for percutaneous and interventional procedures

Interventional breast procedures are guided by the clinical examination or image-detected nonpalpable breast abnormalities to characterize the lesion histologically and plan therapeutic management [11]. Clinical guidance may be sufficient in palpable lesions, but image-guided biopsy allows more precise acquisition with high diagnostic accuracy. Ultrasound-guided procedures are accessible without needing ionizing radiation or intravenous contrast but are rather minimally invasive and less expensive than surgical biopsies [42].

Training and accreditation of surgeon-performed US are essential steps for increasing the use of percutaneous biopsy to diagnose breast pathologies, avoiding additional surgeries and diagnostic delays, particularly in resource constraint settings. Breast surgeons, who perform the percutaneous biopsy, must understand its indications, have technical skills for performing them, and be experienced operators to avoid misleading and harmful procedures, resulting in missed cancer. They should record complications and adverse events during ultrasound-guided interventional procedures and regularly review them to recognize circumstances and opportunities to improve patient management quality. In the same way, surgeons should monitor false-negative rates and inadequate tissue samples of these interventional procedures to audit their practice [9].

US-Guided interventional procedures include fine-needle aspiration cytology (PAAF), core needle biopsy (CNB), vacuum-assisted needle biopsy, placement of brachytherapy devices, and breast tissue ablation.

7.1 US-guided fine-needle aspiration cytology (US-FNAC)

FNAC uses a disposable needle (usually 18 to 27- gauge) connected to a vacuum syringe. It is technically simple, widely available, and easy to plan in outpatient clinics. It can be performed with a low risk of complications. It is an accurate technique and affordable in resource constraints settings [43]. Quality depends on the aspirator's competence and the pathologist's proficiency and expertise in determining its interpretation. FNAC is more appropriate for patients on anticoagulants for lesions adjacent to the skin, close to the chest wall or close to vessels, or patients with implants, or with very small lesions and those with small/thin breasts [44].

Ultrasound-guided needle aspiration puncture is mainly recommended for the aspiration of simple symptomatic cysts. If the aspiration fluid is clear, yellow, greenish-black (no atypical features), it can be discarded and not require further evaluation [45]. In case that the fluid is bloody, it must be sent for cytological analysis. If it looked purulent, it must be sent for culture and gram stain. If suspicious, atypical, or mucin results are found in cytology, re-biopsy or excision of the lesion should be performed. The patient should accomplish a follow-up ultrasound in 4 to 6 weeks when the cyst has been completely evacuated. Whether the cyst recurs, the re-biopsy of the lesion is mandatory [46].

Although core needle biopsy is currently advocated as the standard procedure in most breast centers in developed countries, FNAC continues to be an acceptable and reliable procedure for diagnosing suspicious breast lesions in low and middle-income countries. Two meta-analyses assessed the accuracy performance of FNAC [46, 47]. The meta-analysis of Yu et al. [48] included 46 studies showing pooled sensitivity of 92.7% and specificity of 94.8%; however, the pooled sensitivity and specificity for eleven studies that reported unsatisfactory samples was 92.0% and 76.8%, respectively. The meta-analysis by Wang et al., [47] compared the sensitivity and specificity of CNB and FNAC in twelve studies; the pooled analysis showed that the sensitivity of CNB is better than that of FNAC (87% vs. 74%). However, the specificity of CNB was similar to that of FNAC (98% vs. 96%).

7.2 Ultrasound-guided core needle biopsy (CB)

Ultrasound-Guided Core Needle Biopsy involves 14G–16G spring-loaded automated needles with an excursion throw that allows small cylinders of tissue (specimen) to be cut and collected within the notch of the needle. The needle is extracted from the breast to recover the breast tissue and then re-inserted for further samples. False-negative rates range from 0% [49] to 9% [50], and underestimation rates range from 3.4–100% in atypical ductal hyperplasia, radial scars, papillary lesions, lobular carcinoma in situ (LCIS), and phyllodes tumors [51].

7.3 US vacuum-assisted biopsy (VAB)

VAB is commanded with suction and a rotating cutter. This device uses needles ranging from 7 G to 12 G. Vacuum aspiration pulls lesion tissue samples for collection into a sampling window without removing the needle from the biopsy site [50]. VAB is commanded with suction and a rotating cutter. This device uses needles ranging from 7 G to 12 G.

Currently, there is an increasing interest in using US-guided vacuum-assisted devices for the complete removal of a probably benign lesion [52, 53], with low rates of residual masses, particularly for lesions <1 cm in size [54]. Additionally, successful excision of intraductal masses has been reported in women with nipple discharge [55].

7.4 Guided ablative techniques

Tumor destruction techniques are by heat (hyperthermia) or by cold (cryotherapy) means. Several technologies using hyperthermia are available: radiofrequency, microwaves, interstitial laser, and electroporation [42]. The percutaneous radiofrequency device utilizes five small radiofrequency-enabled wires deploy from the wand (capture basket) to circumscribe the lesion. Radiofrequency passes through the expanded basket, sectioning and coagulating the breast tissue. The device can remove entire lesions up to 25–30 mm [56].

Cryotherapy involves the use of argon gas to generate an ice sphere around the lesion. Ultrasound is used in real-time to visualize the growth of the ice ball around the lesion; this is an outpatient procedure that can be performed under local anesthesia [2].

7.5 Indications for excisional biopsy

Currently, the percutaneous imaging-guided biopsy is the standard for the diagnosis of most breast lesions. However, there are still indications when excisional surgical biopsy should be recommended. The acquaintance of such indications is essential to adopt the multidisciplinary approach and provide the best patient care.

Adequate radiology/histology/clinical correlation is essential, in addition to the cautious post-biopsy surveillance for immediate detection of false-negative results, to prevent delays in cancer diagnosis. Clinical situations where open excisional biopsy should be recommended include [57]:

- Discordance between imaging findings and histopathology.
- Suspicious interval changes in a lesion previously diagnosed as benign pathology.
- High-Risk Lesions: Atypical Ductal Hyperplasia; Lobular carcinoma in Situ; Atypical Lobular Hyperplasia.
- Flat epithelial atypia, radial scar, or radial sclerosing lesion.
- Papillary lesions with atypia. Columnar alteration with cytologic atypia.
- Lesions not amenable to percutaneous biopsies include lesions close to the chest wall or immediately adjacent to the implant, inadequate breast tissue, patient intolerance to lie flat, and lesions superficially located within the skin.
- Lack of adequate retrieval of calcifications (as judged by the radiologist) when calcifications are targeted.

8. Preoperative evaluation of the breast in diagnosed breast cancer

The tumor size obtained by imaging is an important factor in the preoperative planning of breast cancer, whether it is the type of surgery or whether it initiates with neoadjuvant chemotherapy (NAC). Thus, mammography has been considered the standard imaging tool for detecting and assessing tumor size. Currently, the high-resolution US and MRI have been included in the diagnostic flowchart to achieve higher sensitivity [56], underscoring the surgeons' need to know the accuracy of each test to attain affordable breast cancer patient care.

Several studies [57–68] assess mammography, US, and MRI accuracy for measuring preoperative tumor size in patients who do not receive neoadjuvant chemotherapy. These studies showed correlations between ultrasonographic tumor size and pathologic tumor size ranging from 0.40 to 0.93, suggesting that breast ultrasound accurately predicts tumor size for those patients.

Although many studies have evaluated the value of preoperative magnetic resonance imaging (MRI) in invasive breast cancer, its role in clinical practice is still controversial, failing to show surgical outcome benefits [69–71]. A meta-analysis by Houssami and colleagues [69], which included 3,112 patients with breast cancer, found a significant increase in mastectomy rates in the MRI group (16.4% and 25.5%, respectively) with the non-MRI group (8.1% and 18.2%, respectively). This meta-analysis failed to show a surgical outcome benefit because there was no difference in re-excision rate following an initial breast-conservation, with 11.6% in the MRI group compared with 11.4% non-MRI group ($P = .87$). The authors suggest that a routine MRI in breast cancer patients could do more harm than good by identifying foci of disease beyond the lumpectomy bed that would have been eradicated by adjuvant radiation. Two prospective randomized trials [70, 71] assessed the effect of MRI on surgical outcomes in patients with breast cancer, with a primary end-point of reoperation rates (re-excision and conversion to mastectomy). The United Kingdom (UK) randomized trial (COMICE) [70] evaluated the role of breast MRI in 1,625 women who had recently been diagnosed with primary breast malignancy. The trial showed no significant difference in the reoperation rate between the MRI group (18.7%) and the non-MRI group (19.3%). A twenty-eight percent increase in mastectomy rates was considered pathologically avoidable in the MRI group. The MONET trial [71] randomized 418 women with a nonpalpable suspicious mammographic or sonographic finding (BIRADS 3 to BIRADS 5 lesion) to receive preoperative MR Imaging versus usual care (mammography and ultrasound followed by biopsy). One hundred sixty-three women were diagnosed with breast cancer. There was a paradoxical increase in the re-excision rate in the MRI group (34%) and no difference in conversion to mastectomy (11%) compared with the re-excision rate in the non-MRI group (12%, P = .008) and conversion to mastectomy (14% $P = .49$).

9. Preoperative evaluation of axilla in diagnosed breast cancer

Ultrasound is the primary imaging technique to evaluate morphological abnormalities in the lymph nodes. It is a moderately sensitive method (between 26 and 80%) and can be very specific (ranges from 88 to 98%) [72, 73] when a morphological sign that indicates alterations is used as a diagnostic criterion such as general shape, the aspect of the cortex, the hilum and vascularization, rather than size [72–74]. A normal axillary lymph node sizes less than 10 mm, has a smooth and well-defined contour with an echogenic hilum (constitutes the majority of the node), and is surrounded by a thin and uniform hypoechoic cortex measuring less than 3 mm [75]. The ultrasound aspects of tumor infiltration in a crescent order of specificity are diffuse cortical thickening (> 3 mm); focal cortical bulge; eccentric cortical thickening; rounded hypoechoic node; partial or complete effacement of the fatty hilum; non-hilar blood flow on color Doppler; partial or total replacement of the node with an ill-defined (or irregular mass) and microcalcifications in the node [76]. The last step of the tumoral infiltration is spread to the perinodal fat [74, 76–78].

Axillary Ultrasound (AUS) and needle biopsy of abnormal-appearing nodes can appropriately allocate a positive predictive value for detecting nodal metastases [79, 80]. The use of ultrasound and biopsy in an abnormal lymph node improves sensitivity (88% vs. 61%), specificity (100% versus 85%), positive predictive value (91% versus 73%), and negative predictive value (100% versus 77%) compared to US alone [73–75]. The approach for identifying axillary metastases in women with T1 or T2 invasive breast cancer ranges from axillary imaging only in patients with suspicious findings (from physical examination of the axilla) [74] to axillary imaging being performed in all patients [5–7]. The identification of axillary disease on preoperative ultrasound was considered a reliable indicator for preoperative identification of axillary metastases, allowing the surgeon to proceed directly to axillary lymph node dissection (ALND) and omission of sentinel lymph nodes biopsy (SNB) [81].

However, the clinical utility of preoperative axillary imaging evaluation in women with T1 or T2 invasive breast cancer has changed with the American College of Surgeons Oncology Group (ACOSOG) Z0011 study [82] and International Breast Cancer Study Group (IBCSG)23–01 [83]. These randomized controlled trials have established that women with clinical T1–2 invasive breast carcinoma and clinically negative axilla with 1–2 positive sentinel lymph nodes (SLNs) can safely spare ALND without impacting overall survival, disease-free survival, or locoregional recurrence. Hence, several studies have attempted to evaluate whether it can manage patients without palpable adenopathy but with positive axillary nodes identified by ultrasound according to Z0011 criteria [84–87]. These studies have reported that between 43% and 51.9% of patients with nodal metastases on imaging had pN1 disease at surgery, suggesting that a cohort of patients with axillary metastases detected by imaging alone can be candidates for the omission of ALND based on minimal nodal disease. Although a considerable percentage of patients with image-detected positive nodes have pN1 disease, multiple abnormal lymph nodes on axillary imaging were associated with a high likelihood of having pN2–3 disease and worse survival [88–90]. Axillary ultrasound seems to be more suited to exclude high axillary burden than quantifying the nodal disease volume in the event of abnormal axillary lymph nodes detected on preoperative axillary imaging.

In patients with clinically abnormal lymph nodes on physical exam, further evaluation of axilla with AUS with/without needle biopsy should consider appropriating to neoadjuvant chemotherapy, given the high nodal pathologic completed response (PCR) rates of 21 to 65% [91, 92]. Studies support the use of SNB for surgical staging of the axilla with false-negative rates of 8.4 to 14.2% [93–95]. Consequently, the de-escalation of axillary surgery for patients with metastatic axilla may not eliminate the need for the axillary US, but it certainly may make its use more selective.

10. Evaluation of the breast after surgical therapy

Breast imaging is a challenge in evaluating postoperative changes in breast cancer breast due to the wide range of imaging changes after surgery and the risk of recurrent disease. Ultrasound findings depending on the type of surgery performed: mastectomy, breast-conserving therapy, and breast reconstruction; whether radiation therapy has been performed; and the period elapsed from the end of treatment. Breast Ultrasound should perform in addition to, not as a replacement for, mammography [96, 97], for women who have undergone breast-conserving surgery and for the surgical site in patients with mastectomy. There are no post-mastectomy imaging guidelines since they are followed clinically with serial physical examinations. In the absence of breast reconstruction, the chest wall, subcutaneous fat, and skin can be evaluated with ultrasonography [98]. Cutaneous recurrence in patients after mastectomy may be palpable superficial mass.

Understanding the postsurgical imaging findings and their correlation is essential to ensure an accurate interpretation and recommendation. The most common changes in US imaging after breast-conserving surgery are:

- Skin thickening (more than 2 mm) and parenchymal edema, characterized by increased echogenicity and reticular enlargement of breast parenchyma (represented by dilated lymphatics or interstitial fluid). Those findings should start reducing six months after completing radiation therapy and returning to normal by two years of surgical treatment [99].

- Postsurgical scar or fibrotic dermal tissue after skin incision. Postsurgical scar appears as a discrete area of architectural distortion or hypoechoic interruption of the normal parenchyma with an irregular shape, not parallel orientation, strong acoustic shadowing, and absent vascularity. Fibrosis increases up to 18 months and then stabilizes. Therefore, after that period, the tissue that enhances the distortion must be considered suspicious, and biopsy should be considered.

- Postoperative fluid collections in the surgical bed have variable echogenicity (hypoechoic, hyperechoic, or anechoic). The anechoic lesions have a thin wall, sometimes with debris or septa. Hematomas may be ill-defined or present as a mass with distal acoustic enhancement or shadowing and internal complex echoes [10]. Postoperative fluid collection decreases by six months, though, in a few patients, these may persist for years [100].

- Fat necrosis appears as hypoechoic or heterogeneous irregular mass, with acoustic shadowing. These findings may be misinterpreted as suspicious for malignancy. Therefore, in this case, correlating mammographic findings and tissue sampling is indicated (**Figure 6**).

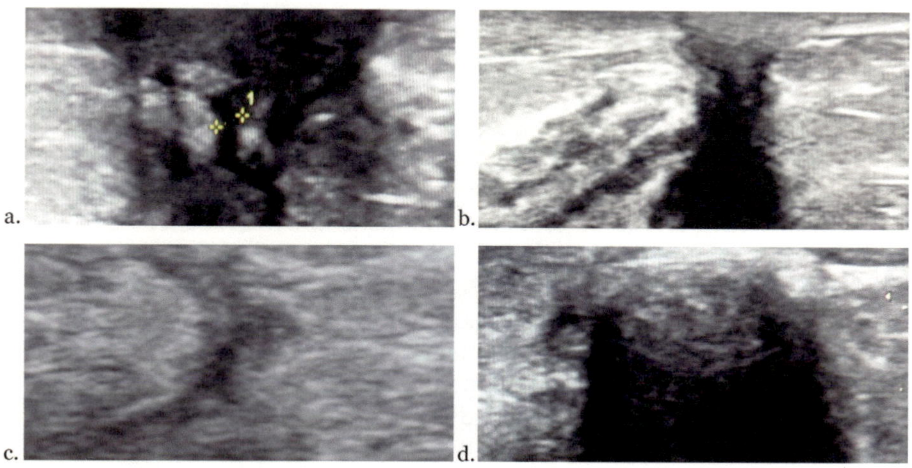

Figure 6.
US Postoperative changes in Breast Conservation Treatment. (a) Parenchymal Edema, represented by reticular enlargement of breast parenchyma with dilated lymphatics (calipers) and interstitial fluid; (b) Postsurgical Scar, a discrete area of hypoechoic distortion with strong acoustic shadowing; (c) Postoperative Fluid Collection in surgical bed; (d) Fat Necrosis: Heterogeneous mass with acoustic shadowing.

11. Evaluation and assessment of the breast after medical therapy

Radiological and clinical evaluation of residual tumor size after neoadjuvant chemotherapy (NAC) is vital for decision-making in breast surgical planning. Physical examination, mammography, and ultrasound are not accurate in assessing the tumor response to NAC. Chagpar et al. [101] examined the accuracy of clinical methods of tumor size assessment (physical examination, mammography, and ultrasound) in evaluating the tumor response to chemotherapy. The correlation coefficients for residual tumor size were estimated for physical examination of 0.42, ultrasound 0.42, and mammography 0.41. Interestingly, clinical measurement estimated by each of these modalities in only 66–75% of cases was within one centimeter of the pathologic tumor size. Likewise, Peintinger et al. [102] showed higher accuracy (89%) with the combination of mammography and sonography in predicting pathological residual tumor size after neoadjuvant chemotherapy, but a moderate agreement (69% of patients) in predicting pathologic tumor size within 0.5 cm.

Therefore, breast ultrasound for clinical evaluation of tumor size is moderately useful for patients receiving chemotherapy first [7]. However, breast MRI has shown an equal or better correlation for these patients and offers the best performance in assessing patients' response and predicting pathological tumor size non-invasively [103, 104].

12. Intraoperative ultrasound (IOUS) in breast surgery

Intraoperative US (IOUS) is a non-invasive procedure that enables the surgeon to perform intraoperative localization and guided excision of a nonpalpable breast lesion, as well as ultrasound-guided operation of traditional palpation-guided surgery [105–109].

Widespread preoperative malignant lesion localization strategies for surgery are wire-guided localization (WGL) and radio occult lesion localization (ROLL)-guided surgery to ensure the whole removal of imaging findings and allow margin clearance [110–112]. Rahusen et al. [110] reported that IOUS (89%) is superior to wire-guided surgery (55%) concerning tumor-free resection margins. A retrospective multicenter study [113] demonstrated that IOUS for nonpalpable invasive breast cancer was more accurate in obtaining adequate margins with the lowest rate of positive margins in the IOUS group (3.7%) than in the wire-localization group (21.3%) and radioguided occult lesion group (25%). Snider et al. showed a reasonable rate of tumor-free resection margins using IOUS (82%) with a smaller excision volume of healthy breast tissue than wire-guided surgery [114].

A meta-analysis [111] of patients with nonpalpable breast cancer treated with IOUS vs. wire-guided localization (WGL) showed that the rate of involved surgical margins for IOUS varies 0–19%. There was a statistically significant difference between IOUS and WGL regarding tumor-free margins favoring IOUS (OR = 0.52; 95%CI: 0.38–0.71). In the meta-analysis of Pan et al. [112], IOUS is an accurate method for localizing nonpalpable and palpable breast cancers by obtaining a high proportion of negative margins and adequate resection volumes in patients undergoing breast-conserving surgery. Thirteen studies were included. Eight were eligible for the impact of IOUS on the margin status of nonpalpable breast cancers; four were suitable for palpable breast cancers, and one was for both nonpalpable and palpable breast cancers. This meta-analysis showed a statistically significant increase in the rate of negative margins using IOUS for both nonpalpable and palpable breast cancers. IOUS-guidance enabled a significantly higher negative margin rate for non-palpable breast cancers than WGL-guidance (RR =1.26, 95% CI =1.09–1.46 from 6 prospective studies; OR = 1.45, 95% CI =0.86–2.43 from 2 retrospective studies). For palpable breast cancers, the relative risk (RR) for IOUS associated negative margins was 2.36 (95% CI =1.26–4.43) in 2 prospective studies, and OR was 2.71 (95% CI = 1.25–5.87) in 2 retrospective studies.

Breast surgeon-performed IOUS-guided excision does not depend on the radiology or nuclear medicine department. This procedure avoids the need for an additional localization procedure preoperatively, is non-stressful for the patients, and allows accurate intraoperative targeting and immediate confirmation of lesion removal with tumor-free margins. The use of this technique allocates hospital resources efficiently in resource-constraint contexts.

IOUS has demonstrated benefits in patients with palpable early-stage primary invasive breast cancer to completely excise the tumor with negative margins and small excision volumes, improving the result. COBALT-trial [107] was a multicenter randomized controlled trial for palpable cancer, comparing IOUS with palpation-guided surgery (PGS). Results of this trial showed a difference in tumor-involved margin of 3% of tumor-involved margins for the invasive component in the IOUS-group compared to 17% in the PGS-group, and thus a significant decrease in additional treatment required in the IOUS group (2% re-excision and 9% boost in IOUS vs. 7% mastectomy, 4% re-excision and 16% boost in the PGS group). Furthermore, secondary results of this trial showed IOUS had smaller odds of having worse cosmetic outcomes than PGS (OR = 0.51, P = 0.045).

Acknowledgements

We would like to thank Darshi Shah for her contribution to the manuscript translation editing.

Conflict of interest

The authors declare no conflict of interest.

Author details

María Eugenia Aponte-Rueda[1*] and María Isabel de Abreu[2]

1 Venezuelan Breast Cancer Research and Education Foundation, Caracas, Venezuela

2 Diagnoimagen Centro Caracas, Caracas, Venezuela

*Address all correspondence to: maruaponte@gmail.com

References

[1] Bennett IC, Biggar MA. The role of ultrasound in the management of breast disease. AJUM 2011; 14 (2): 25-28. DOI: 10.1002/j.2205-0140.2011.tb00191.x

[2] Thompson M, Klimberg VS. Use of ultrasound in breast surgery. Surg Clin N Am 2007; 87:469-484. DOI: 10.1016/j.suc.2007.02.002.

[3] Ahmed M, Abdullah N, Cawthorn S, Usiskin SI, Douek M. Why should breast surgeons use ultrasound? Breast Cancer Res Treat 2014;145(1):1-4. DOI: 10.1007/s10549-014-2926-6.

[4] The American College of Surgeons Ultrasound Examinations by Surgeons [Internet]. 1998. Available at https://www.facs.org/about-acs/statements/31-ultrasound-exam [Accessed 2021-06-24]

[5] ACR practice parameter for the performance of breast ultrasound examination. [Internet]. 2016. Available at https://www.acr.org/-/media/ACR/Files/Practice-Parameters/US-Breast.pdf [Accessed 2021-06-24]

[6] The American Society of Breast Surgeons Performance and Practice Guidelines for Breast Ultrasound [Internet]. 2012. Available from: https://www.breastsurgeons.org/docs/statements/Performance-and-Practice-Guidelines-for-Breast-Ultrasound.pdf [Accessed 2021-06-24]

[7] Evans A, Trimboli RM, Athanasiou A, et al. Breast ultrasound: recommendations for information to women and referring physicians by the European Society of Breast Imaging. Insights Imaging 2018;9(4):449-461. DOI: 10.1007/s13244-018-0636-z.

[8] Kelly KM, Dean J, Comulada W, Lee SJ. Breast Cancer detection using automated whole breast ultrasound and mammography in radiographically dense breast. Eur Radiol 2010;20(3):734-742. DOI: 10.1007/s00330-009-1588-y

[9] D'Orsi CJ, Sickles EA, Mendelson EB, et al. ACR BI-RADS® Atlas: Breast Imaging Reporting and Data System. 5th ed. Reston, VA: American College of Radiology; 2014. 689p.

[10] Mendelson EB, Bohm-Velez M, Berg WA, et al. ACR BI-RADS® Ultrasound. In: ACR BI-RADS® Atlas: Breast Imaging Reporting and Data System. 5th ed. Reston, VA: American College of Radiology; 2014. p 3-149.

[11] Maxwell AJ, Ridley NT, Rubin G, et al. The Royal College of Radiologists Breast Group breast imaging classification. Clin Radiol 2009;64(6):624-627. DOI: 10.1016/j.crad.2009.01.010

[12] Berg WA, Blume JD, Cormack JB, et al. Combined screening with ultrasound and mammography vs. mammography alone in women at elevated risk of breast cancer. JAMA 2008;299(18):2151-63. DOI: 10.1001/jama.299.18.2151

[13] Perry N, Broeders M, de Wolf C, et al. European guidelines for quality assurance in breast cancer screening and diagnosis. Fourth edition--summary document. Ann Oncol 2008;19(4):614-622. DOI: 10.1093/annonc/mdm481

[14] Sung JS. High-quality breast ultrasonography. Radiol Clin North Am 2014;52(3):519-526. DOI: 10.1016/j.rcl.2014.02.012

[15] Gordon PB, Gagnon FA, Lanzkowsky L. Solid breast masses diagnosed as fibroadenoma at fine-needle aspiration biopsy: acceptable rates of growth at long-term follow-up.

Radiology 2003;229(1):233-238. DOI: 10.1148/radiol.2291010282

[16] Barr RG. Future of breast elastography. Ultrasonography 2019; 38(2):93-105. DOI: 10.14366/usg.18053

[17] Lippa N, Hurtevent-Labrot G, Ferron S, Boisserie-Lacroix M. Nipple discharge: The role of imaging. Diagn Interv Imaging 2015;96(10):1017-1032. DOI: 10.1016/j.diii.2015.07.004

[18] Cabioglu N, Hunt KK, Singletary SE, et al. Surgical decision making and factors determining a diagnosis of breast carcinoma in women presenting with nipple discharge. J Am Coll Surg 2003;196(3):354-364. DOI: 10.1016/S1072-7515(02)01606-X

[19] Lang JE, Kuerer HM. Breast ductal secretions: clinical features, potential uses, and possible applications. Cancer Control 2007;14(4):350-359. DOI: 10.1177/107327480701400405

[20] Lorenzon M, Zuiani C, Linda A, et al. Magnetic resonance imaging in patients with nipple discharge: should we recommend it? Eur Radiol 2011;21(5):899-907. DOI: 10.1007/s00330-010-2009-y

[21] Sardanelli F, Boetes C, Borisch B, et al. Magnetic resonance imaging of the breast: recommendations from the EUSOMA working group. Eur J Cancer 2010;46(8):1296-1316. DOI: 10.1016/j.ejca.2010.02.015

[22] Bahl M, Baker JA, Greenup RA, Ghate SV. Diagnostic Value of Ultrasound in Female Patients With Nipple Discharge. AJR Am J Roentgenol 2015;205(1):203-208. DOI: 10.2214/AJR.14.13354

[23] Park CJ, Kim EK, Moon HJ, Yoon JH, Kim MJ. Reliability of Breast Ultrasound BI-RADS Final Assessment in Mammographically Negative Patients with Nipple Discharge and Radiologic Predictors of Malignancy. J Breast Cancer 2016;19(3):308-315. DOI: 10.4048/jbc.2016.19.3.308

[24] Yoon JH, Yoon H, Kim EK, et al. Ultrasonographic evaluation of women with pathologic nipple discharge. Ultrasonography 2017;36(4):310-320. DOI: 10.14366/usg.17013

[25] King TA, Carter KM, Bolton JS, Fuhrman GM. A simple approach to nipple discharge. Am Surg 2000;66(10):960-965.

[26] Gioffrè Florio M, Manganaro T, Pollicino A, Scarfo P, Micali B. Surgical approach to nipple discharge: a ten-year experience. J Surg Oncol 1999;71(4): 235-238. DOI: 10.1002/(sici)1096-9098(199908)71:4<235::aid-jso5>3.0.co;2-#

[27] Morrogh M, Park A, Elkin EB, King TA. Lessons learned from 416 cases of nipple discharge of the breast. Am J Surg 2010;200(1):73-80. DOI: 10.1016/j.amjsurg.2009.06.021

[28] Adepoju LJ, Chun J, El-Tamer M, et al. The value of clinical characteristics and breast-imaging studies in predicting a histopathologic diagnosis of cancer or high-risk lesion in patients with spontaneous nipple discharge. Am J Surg 2005;190(4):644-646. DOI: 10.1016/j.amjsurg.2005.06.032

[29] Sharma R, Dietz J, Wright H, et al. Comparative analysis of minimally invasive microductectomy versus major duct excision in patients with pathologic nipple discharge. Surgery 2005;(4):591-6. DOI: 10.1016/j.surg.2005.07.015

[30] Ashfaq A, Senior D, Pockaj BA, et al. Validation study of a modern treatment algorithm for nipple discharge. Am J Surg 2014;208(2):222-227. DOI: 10.1016/j.amjsurg.2013.12.035

[31] Sabel MS, Helvie MA, Breslin T, et al. Is duct excision still necessary for all cases of suspicious nipple discharge?

Breast J 2012;18(2):157-162. DOI: 10.1111/j.1524-4741.2011.01207.x

[32] Lepori D. Inflammatory breast disease: The radiologist's role. Diagn Interv Imaging 2015;96(10):1045-1064. DOI: 10.1016/j.diii.2015.07.006

[33] Kasales CJ, Han B, Smith JS Jr, et al. Nonpuerperal mastitis and subareolar abscess of the breast. AJR Am J Roentgenol 2014;202(2):W133-W139. DOI: 10.2214/AJR.13.10551

[34] Trop I, Dugas A, David J, et al. Breast abscesses: evidence-based algorithms for diagnosis, management, and follow-up. Radiographics 2011;31(6):1683-1699. DOI: 10.1148/rg.316115521

[35] Ocal K, Dag A, Turkmenoglu O, et al. Granulomatous mastitis: clinical, pathological features, and management. Breast J 2010;16(2):176-182. DOI: 10.1111/j.1524-4741.2009.00879.x

[36] Yilmaz E, Lebe B, Usal C, Balci P. Mammographic and sonographic findings in the diagnosis of idiopathic granulomatous mastitis. Eur Radiol 2001;11(11):2236-2240. DOI: 10.1007/s003300100965

[37] Giess CS, Raza S, Birdwell RL. Distinguishing breast skin lesions from superficial breast parenchymal lesions: diagnostic criteria, imaging characteristics, and pitfalls. Radiographics 2011;31(7):1959-1972. DOI: 10.1148/rg.317115116

[38] Headon H, Kasem A, Mokbel K. Capsular Contracture after Breast Augmentation: An Update for Clinical Practice. Arch Plast Surg 2015;42(5):532-543. DOI: 10.5999/aps.2015.42.5.532

[39] Gossner J. Sonography in capsular contracture after breast augmentation: value of established criteria, new techniques and directions for research. J Ultrasound 2016;20(1):87-89. DOI: 10.1007/s40477-016-0225-2

[40] Lake E, Ahmad S, Dobrashian R. The sonographic appearances of breast implant rupture. Clin Radiol 2013;68(8):851-858. DOI: 10.1016/j.crad.2013.03.014

[41] Expert Panel on Breast Imaging. ACR Appropriateness Criteria® Breast Implant Evaluation. J Am Coll Radiol 2018;15(5S):S13-S25. DOI: 10.1016/j.jacr.2018.03.009

[42] Plantade R. Interventional radiology: the corner-stone of breast management. Diagn Interv Imaging 2013; 94(6):575-591. DOI: 10.1016/j.diii.2013.02.012

[43] Moschetta M, Telegrafo M, Carluccio DA, et al. Comparison between fine needle aspiration cytology (FNAC) and core needle biopsy (CNB) in the diagnosis of breast lesions. G Chir 2014;35(7-8):171-176.

[44] Willems SM, van Deurzen CH, van Diest PJ. Diagnosis of breast lesions: fine-needle aspiration cytology or core needle biopsy? A review. J Clin Pathol 2012;65(4):287-292. DOI: 10.1136/jclinpath-2011-200410

[45] Rinaldi P, Ierardi C, Costantini M, et al. Cystic breast lesions: sonographic findings and clinical management. J Ultrasound Med 2010;29(11):1617-1626. DOI: 10.7863/jum.2010.29.11.1617

[46] Berg WA, Sechtin AG, Marques H, Zhang Z. Cystic breast masses and the ACRIN 6666 experience. Radiol Clin North Am 2010;48(5):931-987. DOI: 10.1016/j.rcl.2010.06.007

[47] Wang M, He X, Chang Y, Sun G, Thabane L. A sensitivity and specificity comparison of fine needle aspiration cytology and core needle biopsy in evaluation of suspicious breast lesions: A systematic review and meta-analysis.

Breast 2017;31:157-166. DOI: 10.1016/j.breast.2016.11.009

[48] Yu YH, Wei W, Liu JL. Diagnostic value of fine-needle aspiration biopsy for breast mass: a systematic review and meta-analysis. BMC Cancer 2012;12:41. DOI: 10.1186/1471-2407-12-41

[49] Liberman L, Feng TL, Dershaw DD, Morris EA, Abramson AF. US-guided core breast biopsy: use and cost-effectiveness. Radiology 1998;208(3):717-723. DOI: 10.1148/radiology.208.3.9722851

[50] Pijnappel RM, van den Donk M, Holland R, et al. Diagnostic accuracy for different strategies of image-guided breast intervention in cases of nonpalpable breast lesions. Br J Cancer 2004;90(3):595-600. DOI: 10.1038/sj.bjc.6601559

[51] O'Flynn EA, Wilson AR, Michell MJ. Image-guided breast biopsy: state-of-the-art. Clin Radiol 2010;65(4):259-270. DOI: 10.1016/j.crad.2010.01.008

[52] Alonso-Bartolomé P, Vega-Bolívar A, Torres-Tabanera M, et al. Sonographically guided 11-G directional vacuum-assisted breast biopsy as an alternative to surgical excision: utility and cost study in probably benign lesions. Acta Radiol 2004;45(4):390-396. DOI: 10.1080/02841850410005633

[53] Kim MJ, Park BW, Kim SI, et al. Long-term follow-up results for ultrasound-guided vacuum-assisted removal of benign palpable breast mass. Am J Surg 2010;199(1):1-7. DOI: 10.1016/j.amjsurg.2008.11.037

[54] Grady I, Gorsuch H, Wilburn-Bailey S. Long-term outcome of benign fibroadenomas treated by ultrasound-guided percutaneous excision. Breast J 2008;14(3):275-278. doi: 10.1111/j.1524-4741.2008.00574.x

[55] Bonaventure T, Cormier B, Lebas P, Bonneau C, Michenet P. Benign papilloma: is US-guided vacuum-assisted breast biopsy an alternative to surgical biopsy? J Radiol 2007;88: 1165-1168. DOI: 10.1016/s0221-0363(07)89928-8

[56] Fine RE, Staren ED. Percutaneous radiofrequency-assisted excision of fibroadenomas. Am J Surg 2006;192(4):545-547. DOI: 10.1016/j.amjsurg.2006.06.011

[57] Liberman L. Clinical management issues in percutaneous core breast biopsy. Radiol Clin North Am 2000;38(4):791-807. DOI: 10.1016/s0033-8389(05)70201-3

[58] Melnikow J, Fenton JJ, Whitlock EP, et al. Supplemental Screening for Breast Cancer in Women With Dense Breasts: A Systematic Review for the U.S. Preventive Service Task Force [Internet]. Rockville (MD): Agency for Healthcare Research and Quality (US); 2016. (Evidence Syntheses, No. 126.) Available from: https://www.ncbi.nlm.nih.gov/books/NBK343793/[Accessed: 2021-06-25]

[59] Hieken TJ, Harrison J, Herreros J, Velasco JM. Correlating sonography, mammography, and pathology in the assessment of breast cancer size. Am J Surg 2001;182(4):351-354. DOI: 10.1016/s0002-9610(01)00726-7

[60] Madjar H, Ladner HA, Sauerbrei W, et al. Preoperative staging of breast cancer by palpation, mammography and high-resolution ultrasound. Ultrasound Obstet Gynecol 1993;3(3):185-190. DOI: 10.1046/j.1469-0705.1993.03030185.x

[61] Bosch AM, Kessels AG, Beets GL, et al. Preoperative estimation of the pathological breast tumour size by physical examination, mammography and ultrasound: a prospective study on 105 invasive tumours. Eur J Radiol

2003;48(3):285-292. DOI: 10.1016/s0720-048x(03)00081-0

[62] Leddy R, Irshad A, Metcalfe A, et al. Comparative accuracy of preoperative tumor size assessment on mammography, sonography, and MRI: Is the accuracy affected by breast density or cancer subtype? J Clin Ultrasound 2016;44(1):17-25. DOI: 10.1002/jcu.22290

[63] Gruber IV, Rueckert M, Kagan KO, et al. Measurement of tumour size with mammography, sonography and magnetic resonance imaging as compared to histological tumour size in primary breast cancer. BMC Cancer 2013;13:328. DOI: 10.1186/1471-2407-13-328

[64] Yang WT, Lam WW, Cheung H, et al. Sonographic, magnetic resonance imaging, and mammographic assessments of preoperative size of breast cancer. J Ultrasound Med 1997;16(12):791-797. DOI: 10.7863/jum.1997.16.12.791

[65] Golshan M, Fung BB, Wiley E, et al. Prediction of breast cancer size by ultrasound, mammography and core biopsy. Breast 2004;13(4):265-271. DOI: 10.1016/j.breast.2004.05.005

[66] Katz B, Raker C, Edmonson D, et al. Predicting Breast Tumor Size for Pre-operative Planning: Which Imaging Modality is Best? Breast J 2017;23(1): 52-58. DOI: 10.1111/tbj.12680

[67] Stein RG, Wollschläger D, Kreienberg R; BRENDA Study Group. The impact of breast cancer biological subtyping on tumor size assessment by ultrasound and mammography - a retrospective multicenter cohort study of 6543 primary breast cancer patients. BMC Cancer 2016;16:459. DOI: 10.1186/s12885-016-2426-7

[68] Cortadellas T, Argacha P, Acosta J, et al. Estimation of tumor size in breast cancer comparing clinical examination, mammography, ultrasound and MRI-correlation with the pathological analysis of the surgical specimen. Gland Surg 2017;6(4):330-335. DOI: 10.21037/gs.2017.03.09

[69] Houssami N, Turner R, Morrow M. Preoperative magnetic resonance imaging in breast cancer: meta-analysis of surgical outcomes. Ann Surg 2013;257(2):249-255. DOI: 10.1097/SLA.0b013e31827a8d17

[70] Turnbull L, Brown S, Harvey I, et al. Comparative effectiveness of MRI in breast cancer (COMICE) trial: a randomised controlled trial. Lancet 2010;375(9714):563-571. DOI: 10.1016/S0140-6736(09)62070-5

[71] Peters NH, van Esser S, van den Bosch MA, et al. Preoperative MRI and surgical management in patients with nonpalpable breast cancer: the MONET - randomised controlled trial. Eur J Cancer 2011;47(6):879-886. DOI: 10.1016/j.ejca.2010.11.035

[72] Bedi DG, Krishnamurthy R, Krishnamurthy S, et al. Cortical morphologic features of axillary lymph nodes as a predictor of metastasis in breast cancer: in vitro sonographic study. AJR Am J Roentgenol 2008;191(3):646-652. DOI: 10.2214/AJR.07.2460

[73] Alvarez S, Añorbe E, Alcorta P, et al. Role of sonography in the diagnosis of axillary lymph node metastases in breast cancer: a systematic review. AJR Am J Roentgenol 2006;186(5):1342-1348. DOI: 10.2214/AJR.05.0936

[74] Abe H, Schmidt RA, Kulkarni K, et al. Axillary lymph nodes suspicious for breast cancer metastasis: sampling with US-guided 14-gauge core-needle biopsy--clinical experience in 100 patients. Radiology 2009;250(1):41-49. DOI: 10.1148/radiol.2493071483

[75] Maxwell F, de Margerie Mellon C, Bricout M, et al. Diagnostic strategy for the assessment of axillary lymph node status in breast cancer. Diagn Interv Imaging 2015 ;96(10):1089-1101. DOI: 10.1016/j.diii.2015.07.007

[76] Ecanow JS, Abe H, Newstead GM, Ecanow DB, Jeske JM. Axillary staging of breast cancer: what the radiologist should know. Radiographics 2013;33(6):1589-1612. DOI: 10.1148/rg.336125060

[77] Mainiero MB. Regional lymph node staging in breast cancer: the increasing role of imaging and ultrasound-guided axillary lymph node fine needle aspiration. Radiol Clin North Am 2010;48(5):989-997. DOI: 10.1016/j.rcl.2010.06.010

[78] Choi YJ, Ko EY, Han BK, et al. High-resolution ultrasonographic features of axillary lymph node metastasis in patients with breast cancer. Breast 2009;18(2):119-122. DOI: 10.1016/j.breast.2009.02.004

[79] Diepstraten SC, Sever AR, Buckens CF, et al. Value of preoperative ultrasound-guided axillary lymph node biopsy for preventing completion axillary lymph node dissection in breast cancer: a systematic review and meta-analysis. Ann Surg Oncol 2014;21(1):51-9. DOI: 10.1245/s10434-013-3229-6

[80] Houssami N, Ciatto S, Turner RM, Cody HS 3rd, Macaskill P. Preoperative ultrasound-guided needle biopsy of axillary nodes in invasive breast cancer: meta-analysis of its accuracy and utility in staging the axilla. Ann Surg 2011;254(2):243-251. DOI: 10.1097/SLA.0b013e31821f1564

[81] Boughey JC, Moriarty JP, Degnim AC, Gregg MS, Egginton JS, Long KH. Cost modeling of preoperative axillary ultrasound and fine-needle aspiration to guide surgery for invasive breast cancer. Ann Surg Oncol 2010;17(4):953-958. doi: 10.1245/s10434-010-0919-1

[82] Giuliano AE, McCall L, Beitsch P, et al. Locoregional recurrence after sentinel lymph node dissection with or without axillary dissection in patients with sentinel lymph node metastases: the American College of Surgeons Oncology Group Z0011 randomized trial. Ann Surg 2010;252(3):426-432. DOI: 10.1097/SLA.0b013e3181f08f32

[83] Galimberti V, Cole BF, Zurrida S, et al. Axillary dissection versus no axillary dissection in patients with sentinel-node micrometastases (IBCSG 23-01): a phase 3 randomised controlled trial. Lancet Oncol 2013;14(4):297-305. DOI: 10.1016/S1470-2045(13)70035-4

[84] Ahmed M, Jozsa F, Baker R, et al. Meta-analysis of tumour burden in pre-operative axillary ultrasound positive and negative breast cancer patients. Breast Cancer Res Treat 2017;166(2):329-336. DOI: 10.1007/s10549-017-4405-3

[85] Pilewskie M, Jochelson M, Gooch JC, et al. Is Preoperative Axillary Imaging Beneficial in Identifying Clinically Node-Negative Patients Requiring Axillary Lymph Node Dissection? J Am Coll Surg 2016;222(2):138-145. DOI: 10.1016/j.jamcollsurg.2015.11.013

[86] Harris CK, Tran HT, Lee K, et al. Positive Ultrasound-guided Lymph Node Needle Biopsy in Breast Cancer may not Mandate Axillary Lymph Node Dissection. Ann Surg Oncol 2017;24(10):3004-3010. DOI: 10.1245/s10434-017-5935-y

[87] Abe H, Schacht D, Sennett CA, Newstead GM, Schmidt RA. Utility of preoperative ultrasound for predicting pN2 or higher stage axillary lymph node involvement in patients with newly diagnosed breast cancer. AJR Am J

Roentgenol 2013;200(3):696-702. DOI: 10.2214/AJR.12.9036

[88] Verheuvel NC, van den Hoven I, Ooms HW, Voogd AC, Roumen RM. The role of ultrasound-guided lymph node biopsy in axillary staging of invasive breast cancer in the post-ACOSOG Z0011 trial era. Ann Surg Oncol 2015;22(2):409-415. DOI: 10.1245/s10434-014-4071-1

[89] Caudle AS, Kuerer HM, Le-Petross HT, et al. Predicting the extent of nodal disease in early-stage breast cancer. Ann Surg Oncol 2014;21(11):3440-3447. DOI: 10.1245/s10434-014-3813-4

[90] van Wely BJ, de Wilt JH, Francissen C, Teerenstra S, Strobbe LJ. Meta-analysis of ultrasound-guided biopsy of suspicious axillary lymph nodes in the selection of patients with extensive axillary tumour burden in breast cancer. Br J Surg 2015;102(3): 159-168. DOI: 10.1002/bjs.9663

[91] Boughey JC, McCall LM, Ballman KV, et al. Tumor biology correlates with rates of breast-conserving surgery and pathologic complete response after neoadjuvant chemotherapy for breast cancer: findings from the ACOSOG Z1071 (Alliance) Prospective Multicenter Clinical Trial. Ann Surg 2014;260(4):608-614. DOI: 10.1097/SLA.0000000000000924.

[92] Hennessy BT, Hortobagyi GN, Rouzier R, et al. Outcome after pathologic complete eradication of cytologically proven breast cancer axillary node metastases following primary chemotherapy. J Clin Oncol 2005;23(36):9304-9311. DOI: 10.1200/JCO.2005.02.5023

[93] Kuehn T, Bauerfeind I, Fehm T, et al. Sentinel-lymph-node biopsy in patients with breast cancer before and after neoadjuvant chemotherapy (SENTINA): a prospective, multicentre cohort study. Lancet Oncol 2013;14(7):609-618. DOI: 10.1016/S1470-2045(13)70166-9

[94] Boughey JC, Suman VJ, Mittendorf EA, et al. Sentinel lymph node surgery after neoadjuvant chemotherapy in patients with node-positive breast cancer: the ACOSOG Z1071 (Alliance) clinical trial. JAMA 2013;310(14):1455-1461. DOI: 10.1001/jama.2013.278932

[95] Boileau JF, Poirier B, Basik M, et al. Sentinel node biopsy after neoadjuvant chemotherapy in biopsy-proven node-positive breast cancer: the SN FNAC study. J Clin Oncol 2015;33(3):258-264. DOI: 10.1200/JCO.2014.55.7827

[96] Khatcheressian JL, Hurley P, Bantug E, et al. Breast cancer follow-up and management after primary treatment: American Society of Clinical Oncology clinical practice guideline update. J Clin Oncol 2013;31(7):961-965. DOI: 10.1200/JCO.2012.45.9859

[97] Expert Panel on Breast Imaging, Lewin AA, Moy L, Baron P, et al. ACR Appropriateness Criteria® Stage I Breast Cancer: Initial Workup and Surveillance for Local Recurrence and Distant Metastases in Asymptomatic Women. J Am Coll Radiol 2019;16(11S): S428-S439. DOI: 10.1016/j.jacr.2019.05.024

[98] Esen G, Olgun DC. Ultrasonography of the Postsurgical Breast Including Implants. Ultrasound Clinics 2008;3: 295-329

[99] Margolis NE, Morley C, Lotfi P, et al. Update on imaging of the postsurgical breast. Radiographics 2014;34(3):642-660. DOI: 10.1148/rg.343135059

[100] Dershaw DD. Breast imaging and the conservative treatment of breast cancer. Radiol Clin North Am 2002;40(3):501-516. DOI: 10.1016/s0033-8389(01)00003-3

[101] Chagpar AB, Middleton LP, Sahin AA, et al. Accuracy of physical examination, ultrasonography, and mammography in predicting residual pathologic tumor size in patients treated with neoadjuvant chemotherapy. Ann Surg 2006;243(2):257-264. DOI: 10.1097/01.sla.0000197714.14318.6f

[102] Peintinger F, Kuerer HM, Anderson K, et al. Accuracy of the combination of mammography and sonography in predicting tumor response in breast cancer patients after neoadjuvant chemotherapy. Ann Surg Oncol 2006;13(11):1443-1449. DOI: 10.1245/s10434-006-9086-9

[103] Marinovich ML, Macaskill P, Irwig L, et al. Meta-analysis of agreement between MRI and pathologic breast tumour size after neoadjuvant chemotherapy. Br J Cancer 2013;109(6):1528-1536. DOI: 10.1038/bjc.2013.473

[104] Hylton NM, Blume JD, Bernreuter WK, et al. Locally advanced breast cancer: MR imaging for prediction of response to neoadjuvant chemotherapy--results from ACRIN 6657/I-SPY TRIAL. Radiology 2012;263(3):663-672. DOI: 10.1148/radiol.12110748

[105] Bennett IC, Greenslade J, Chiam H. Intraoperative ultrasound-guided excision of nonpalpable breast lesions. World J Surg 2005;29(3):369-374. DOI: 10.1007/s00268-004-7554-6

[106] Rahusen FD, Bremers AJ, Fabry HF, et al. Ultrasound-guided lumpectomy of nonpalpable breast cancer versus wire-guided resection: a randomized clinical trial. Ann Surg Oncol 2002;9(10):994-998. DOI: 10.1007/BF02574518

[107] Krekel NM, Haloua MH, Lopes Cardozo AM, et al. Intraoperative ultrasound guidance for palpable breast cancer excision (COBALT trial): a multicentre, randomised controlled trial. Lancet Oncol 2013;14(1):48-54. DOI: 10.1016/S1470-2045(12)70527-2

[108] Ngô C, Pollet AG, Laperrelle J, et al. Intraoperative ultrasound localization of nonpalpable breast cancers. Ann Surg Oncol 2007;14(9):2485-2489. DOI: 10.1245/s10434-007-9420-x

[109] Ivanovic NS, Zdravkovic DD, Skuric Z, et al. Optimization of breast cancer excision by intraoperative ultrasound and marking needle - technique description and feasibility. World J Surg Oncol 2015;13:153. DOI: 10.1186/s12957-015-0568-8

[110] Rahusen FD, Bremers AJ, Fabry HF, et al. Ultrasound-guided lumpectomy of nonpalpable breast cancer versus wire-guided resection: a randomized clinical trial. Ann Surg Oncol 2002;9(10): 994-998. DOI: 10.1007/BF02574518

[111] Ahmed M, Douek M. Intra-operative ultrasound versus wire-guided localization in the surgical management of nonpalpable breast cancers: systematic review and meta-analysis. Breast Cancer Res Treat 2013;140(3): 435-446. DOI: 10.1007/s10549-013-2639-2

[112] Pan H, Wu N, Ding H, et al. Intraoperative ultrasound guidance is associated with clear lumpectomy margins for breast cancer: a systematic review and meta-analysis. PLoS One 2013;8(9):e74028. DOI: 10.1371/journal.pone.0074028

[113] Krekel NM, Zonderhuis BM, Stockmann HB, et al. A comparison of three methods for nonpalpable breast cancer excision. Eur J Surg Oncol 2011;37(2):109-115. DOI: 10.1016/j.ejso.2010.12.006

[114] Snider HC Jr, Morrison DG. Intraoperative ultrasound localization of nonpalpable breast lesions. Ann Surg Oncol 1999;6(3):308-314. DOI: 10.1007/s10434-999-0308-9

Chapter 7

Accuracy and Efficacy of Ultrasound-Guided Pes Anserinus Bursa Injection

Jong Hwa Lee, Jae Uk Lee and Seung Wan Yoo

Abstract

The term "pes anserinus tendinobursitis (PATB)" is generally used to describe the inflammatory condition of pes anserinus bursa (PAB). Ultrasound (US) is widely used as a diagnostic and therapeutic tool to improve the assessment and management of joints and soft tissues. We performed the study to prove the accuracy and efficacy of US-guided injections in patients with PATB by comparing blind interventions. Forty-seven patients were randomly assigned to an US-guided and a blind injection group. The patients in the US-guided group were given injections under sonographic visualization. Otherwise, in the blind group, injections were provided in the conventional technique without any sonographic guidance. After the management, the accuracy of the injections was assessed by identifying the injectate location using the US. Treatment efficacy was evaluated using the visual analog scale (VAS) of knee tenderness. The US-guided group showed that the injectates were located at the PAB accurately in all participants, whereas the blind group revealed that the materials were found to be at the bursa side only in 4 out of 22 patients. VAS scores of the US-guided group significantly improved compared to the blind group. In conclusion, US-guided PAB injections are more accurate and efficacious than blind approaches.

Keywords: pes anserinus tendinobursitis, bursa injection, ultrasound

1. Introduction

The pes anserinus (PA), which means "Goose foot" in Latin, consists of the conjoined tendon of the sartorius, gracilis, and semitendinosus muscles. It inserts into the proximal anteromedial aspect of the tibia approximately 5 cm distal to the medial tibial joint line. Biomechanically, it provides secondary restraint against valgus forces of the knee joint [1–4]. The PA bursa (PAB) is located deep to the PA tendon and serves to reduce friction between three tendons and the deep structures including the tibia and the medial collateral ligament (MCL). Commonly, it does not communicate with the knee joint space [3].

The first description of the region in literature dates back to 1937. Moschcowitz described knee pain almost exclusively in women who complained of pain when going downstairs or upstairs, or had difficulty in getting up from a chair, or flexing their knees [5]. PA bursitis or tendinitis, or also called PA tendinobursitis (PATB), is usually used to describe the inflammatory condition of the PAB mainly caused by repetitive friction over the bursa or by direct trauma. It can be observed in patients with rheumatoid arthritis, osteoarthritis (OA), and diabetes mellitus. The risk increases in people who are obese or have valgus knee deformity [6–8]. PATB is clinically common in obese female OA patients. The distinction between PA bursitis and tendinitis is difficult because of the proximity of the structures. In addition, its pathology remains unknown and is still controversial. However, the treatment strategy is similar for those conditions [9].

The exact prevalence of PATB is unknown. It has been reported at a wide range of levels, between 2.5 and 70% [10]. Frequently, the incidence tended to be underestimated due to difficulty in diagnosis. In a retrospective review of 509 knee MRIs obtained on 488 patients with suspected "internal derangement" at an orthopedic outpatient clinic, a 2.5% prevalence of PATB was detected [11]. Sometimes, fluid collection in semimembranosus bursa, around the collateral ligament, or meniscal cyst can make the differential diagnosis difficult. Therefore, it was suggested that fluid collection in the PA bursa accompanied by clinical symptoms such as pain in the medial side of the knee was helpful for diagnosis. In a prospective study, a total of 170 knees of 85 patients with OA were assessed with the US, and the incidence of PA bursitis was 20% [12]. They presented that PA bursitis was more common in women and at advanced ages and was observed in one of every symptomatic OA patient.

The clinical diagnosis of PATB is based on symptoms, including pain in the medial aspect of the knee when going downstairs or upstairs, morning pain and rigidity for more than 1 h, sensitivity to compression on the tendon insertion area, and occasional local edema [11]. Resolving the pain after a local anesthetic injection may also be helpful for diagnosis [12]. MRI can be useful in the diagnosis of PATB when swelling, fluid collection associated with the inflammatory process are observed as like most of the soft tissue pathologies. The exam can be a good method to detect and differentiate cystic lesion within and around the knee [13]. However, results of the image often do not allow to identify structures that are responsible for the symptoms of PATB.

2. Significance of US-guided injections

Many studies have researched the accuracy and efficacy of US-guided injections compared to blind (without a guide) techniques. Gilliland et al. [14] presented a systemic review about the efficacy of US-guided intra-articular and periarticular injection compared with anatomic standard injection using palpation/anatomic landmarks in the joints of the knee, shoulder, foot, ankle, wrist, and hand. They concluded that accuracy was improved with the use of US-guided injection and short-term outcome improvements were found in the US-guided groups. Berkoff et al. [15] reviewed the clinical utility of US-guided intra-articular knee injections in comparison with palpation-guided anatomical injections. The study suggested that US guidance significantly improved the accuracy of injection in the target joint space. The accuracy induced the improvement of clinical outcomes and cost-effectiveness.

PAB injection is usually performed by a blind method in actual clinical settings because the structure locates close to the superficial layer relative to the shoulder or knee joint. Therefore, it has not been sufficiently studied in relation to the ultrasound (US) guidance. Finnoff et al. [10] compared the accuracy of US-guided and unguided PAB injections in 24 cadaveric lower extremities specimens. The accuracy rate was 92% in the US-guided group and 17% in the unguided group. In spite of the superficial location, most unguided PAB injections failed to place the injectate within the bursa, while US-guided injection showed a high degree of accuracy. Because it was a study using cadavers, therapeutic efficacy in clinical conditions could not be identified. The exact pathology of PATB is still not completely known, which has been studied for more than 80 years. Furthermore, the injection location to prove its effect has not been sufficiently investigated.

This study was conducted with the aim of assessing the accuracy of US-guided PAB injections and evaluating the clinical outcomes of the efficacy of injection by comparing them to blind injections. The study also examined whether the location of injectate could suggest the main source of pain.

3. Methods and materials

3.1 Participants

Patients who were clinically diagnosed with PATB were recruited. Symptoms were determined to include medial knee pain when going downstairs or upstairs, rigidity for more than 1 h, sensitivity to compression on the tendon insertion area, and occasional local edema. All participants were randomly assigned into two groups—the US-guided injection group and the blind injection group. The randomization and allocation sequences were generated by using Microsoft Excel. Seven patients were dropped out to follow-up, and a total of 47 patients were finally analyzed (**Figure 1**). Patients who had knee OA (grade I–III Kellgren-Lawrence), pain in the medial aspect of the knee, and symptoms lasting for at least 3 months were included. These patients presented maximal tenderness over the PAB, not on the joint line or around the patella bone. The exclusion criteria were history of traumatic injury or mechanical derangement, surgical intervention, systemic inflammatory disorders, concomitant severe rheumatic disease, microcrystalline arthropathy, or fibromyalgia.

The study was carried out with permission from the institutional review board of our hospital. Informed consent was obtained from each subject for study participation, according to the ethical guidelines of the hospital after the subject fully understood the study's purpose and methodology.

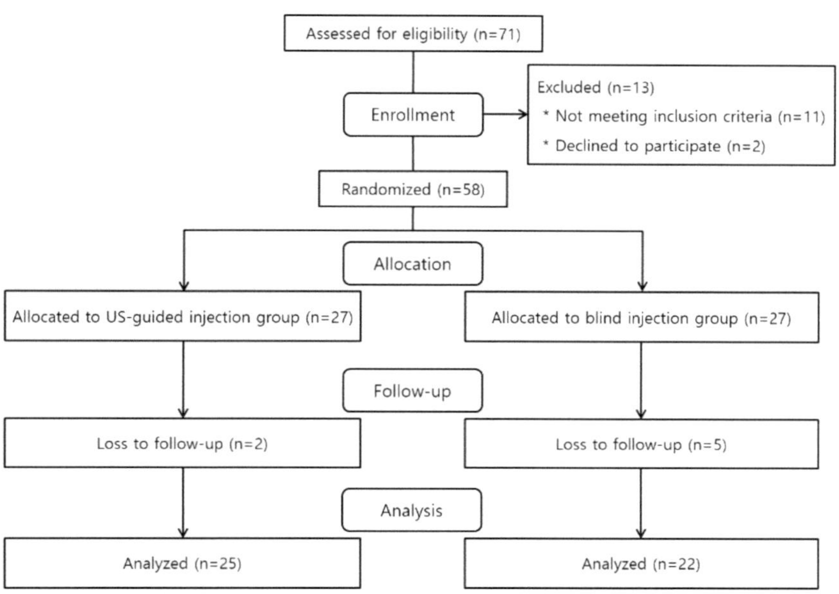

Figure 1.
Study flowchart.

3.2 US-guided injection technique

All sonographic examinations and injections were performed by one expert physician with over 10 years of experience in the musculoskeletal US and managing knee OA. In the preparation, the subjects were placed in the supine position with the knee flexed 5-10 degrees. After marking the PAB area, the skin was prepped with the usual products. US assessment was performed on the medial part of the knee using a linear array probe with a 6–12-MHz frequency and penetration depths of 2.5–4 cm. The needle was inserted at the point where the PA crossed over the anterior fibers of the MCL. The transducer was positioned in a longitudinal orientation relative to the anterior fibers of the MCL, with an oblique transverse orientation relative to the PA. Under US guidance, a 25-gauge 38-mm needle was inserted through the skin proximal to the transducer in a longitudinal plane. Continuously advanced in the distal direction and introduced the needle tip into the tissue space between the PA and the MCL. When the needle tip was visualized between the middle of the PA and the MCL, the materials were injected under direct sonographic visualization (**Figures 2** and **3**).

3.3 Blind injection technique

The same physician who carried out US-guided injections provided the blind injections. The blind injection was performed in a similar technique to the method described previously [16]. The subjects were placed in the supine position, with the slightly flexed knee as like for the US-guided methods; palpated the point of maximal tenderness and marked it; prepped the skin using a usual product; inserted the 25-gauge 38-mm needle to the skin perpendicularly into the maximal tender point until touching the bone gently. After that, the needle of 2–3 mm is withdrawn to avoid injecting into the conjoined tendon directly; the materials are injected into the syringe, which should easily flow.

3.4 Injection material

The injection material was a mixture of 20 mg of triamcinolone acetonide and 1 mL of 1% lidocaine. It was injected at the maximal tender point in the PAB area

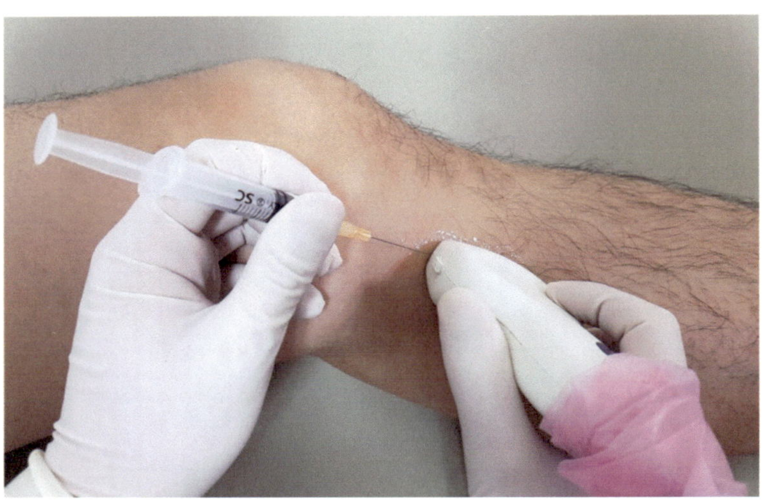

Figure 2.
US-guided injection, the transducer was positioned in a longitudinal orientation relative to the anterior fibers of the medial collateral ligament, with an oblique transverse orientation relative to the pes anserinus.

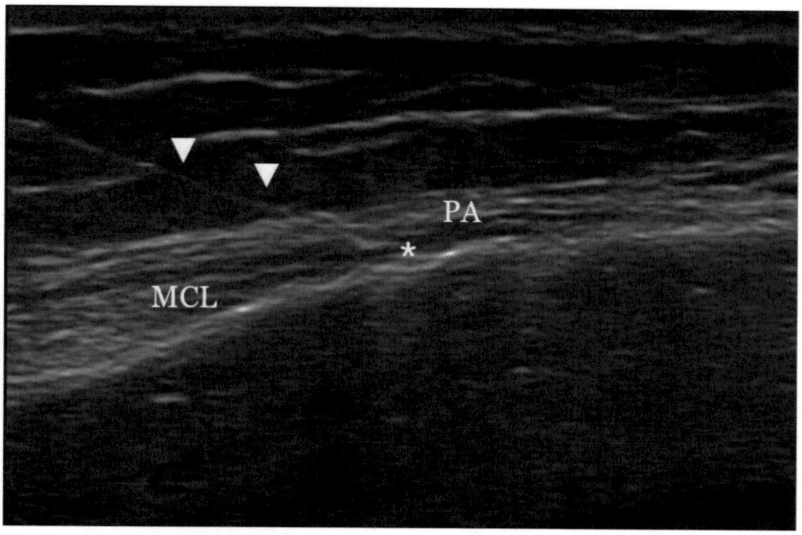

Figure 3.
US-guided injection, longitudinal ultrasound image of a needle (arrowhead) in the pes anserinus bursa (asterisk) between the medial collateral ligament (MCL) and the pes anserinus (PA) tendon.

under US guidance and blind method each. After the PA injections, to identify the location of the material, sonographic scanning was performed in both groups.

3.5 Assessment

After the management, the accuracy of the injections was assessed by identifying the injectate location using the US. The injectate location was evaluated by a second operator who was unaware of the previous procedure with more than 8 years of musculoskeletal US experience in diagnosis and management.

Treatment efficacy to the injection was assessed with a pain visual analog scale (VAS) of knee tenderness. The patients were asked to check the degree of pain intensity ranging from 0 (the absence of pain) to 10 (the worst pain ever). Because all the participants in this study had degenerative arthritis of the knees, it was important to distinguish between articular pain and bursal pain. If the patients described it as simply knee pain, the distinction could be confusing. Therefore, the VAS scores were measured while the constant force was applied to the tender point of PA by an examiner with a pressure algometer (FPK-5®Wagner Instruments, USA). This measurement was performed before 1 week and 4 weeks after the injection.

We did not provide any drugs which had the analgesic effect, including non-steroidal anti-inflammatory drugs that could mask the pain symptoms of the participants. All patients were informed about discomforts after injection. To avoid possible tendon tear or rupture, the patients were advised to rest for at least 2–3 days with the application of ice 3 times every day. Also, they were taught not to do jumping, squatting, kneeling, and bending of the knee for 3 weeks. About 4 weeks after the procedures, complications that had occurred were assessed by individual interviews.

The data were analyzed by using Windows SPSS 18.0 software. To evaluate the outcome measurements before and after treatment in each group, the Wilcoxon signed-rank test was used. Statistical processing was conducted with the Mann-Whitney *U* test for comparison between the two groups. A statistical significance level was set at $p < 0.05$.

4. Results

Forty-seven patients diagnosed with PATB and knee OA were finally recruited. The US-guided injection group included 25 patients with a mean age of 65.36 ± 7.12 years (two men and 23 women). The blind injection group included 22 patients with a mean age of 63.40 ± 6.20 years (two men and 20 women). There were no significant differences in general characteristics including knee OA K-L grade, and baseline VAS scores between the two groups (**Table 1**).

In the US-guided injection group, changes of the VAS for PA tenderness showed that pain reduced significantly from 6.82 ± 1.45 at baseline to 2.28 ± 1.08 1 week after the injection and 3.27 ± 0.94 4 weeks after the injection ($p < 0.05$) (**Table 2**). In the blind injection group, changes of the VAS also revealed that pain reduced statistically from 6.45 ± 1.12 at baseline to 3.95 ± 1.23 1 week after the injection and 4.60 ± 0.95 4 weeks after the injection ($p < 0.05$) (**Table 2**).

Table 3 shows the comparison between the two groups in changes of the VAS score for PA tenderness. The US-guided injection group showed that pain reduced significantly greater than the blind group with regard to ΔVAS scores at 1 week after injection (4.54 ± 0.98 vs. 2.50 ± 1.03) and 4 weeks after injection (3.55 ± 1.14 vs. 1.85 ± 0.84).

After the PAB injections, the injectates were found to be accurate in the PAB, between the PA tendon and the tibia or the MCL, in all 25 subjects in the US-guided injection group (**Figure 4**). On the other hand, in the blind injection group the materials were found to be located in the PAB in only four of 22 subjects, deep to the MCL in two, and superficial to the PA tendon in 16 patients (**Figure 5**). Most injectates were administered outside the PA bursa.

	US-guided group	Blind group	p value
Age (year)	65.36 ± 7.12	63.40 ± 6.20	0.412
Sex (male/female)	2/23	2/20	
Right/left	11/14	12/10	
Knee OA duration (year)	7.21 ± 6.33	6.35 ± 6.24	0.137
Knee OA K-L grade	2.20 ± 0.56	2.15 ± 0.57	0.652
Baseline pain score			
VAS (knee pain)	5.24 ± 1.20	4.80 ± 1.45	0.255
VAS (PA tenderness)	6.82 ± 1.45	6.45 ± 1.12	0.320

Values are presented as mean ± standard deviation.
US = ultrasound; OA = osteoarthritis; K-L grade = Kellgren-Lawrence grade; VAS = visual analog scale; PA = pes anserinus.

Table 1.
Baseline characteristics of both groups.

VAS	US-guided group	Blind group
Baseline	6.82 ± 1.45	6.45 ± 1.12
1 week after injection	2.28 ± 1.08*	3.95 ± 1.23*
4 weeks after injection	3.27 ± 0.94*	4.60 ± 0.95*

Values are presented as mean ± standard deviation.
VAS = visual analog scale; PA = pes anserinus; US = ultrasound.
**$p < 0.05$ by Wilcoxon signed-rank test.*

Table 2.
Changes of VAS of PA tenderness comparing baseline.

Intra-tendon injection was not performed on any of the participants in either group. Complications were not reported after the intervention in both groups.

	US-guided group	Blind group	p value
ΔVAS			
1 week after injection	4.54 ± 0.98	2.50 ± 1.03	0.000*
4 weeks after injection	3.55 ± 1.14	1.85 ± 0.84	0.003*

Values are presented as mean ± standard deviation.
VAS = visual analog scale; US = ultrasound.
**p < 0.05 by Mann-Whitney U test.*

Table 3.
Changes of VAS of PA tenderness between two groups.

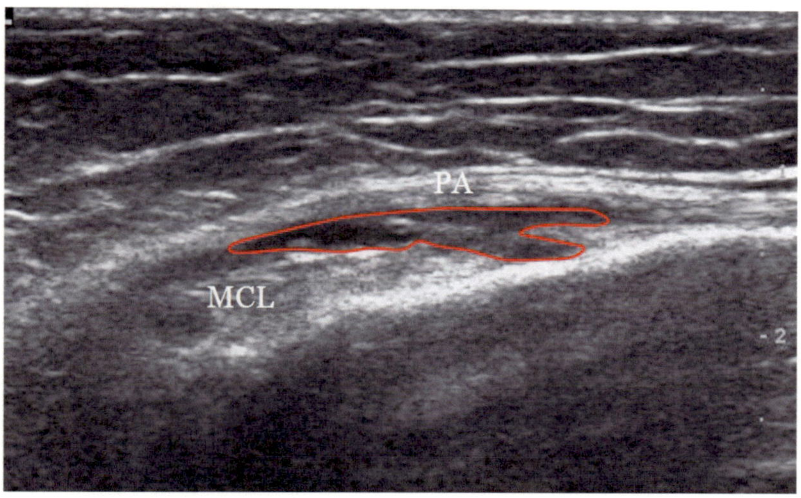

Figure 4.
Ultrasound image of the injectate location after injection; intra-pes anserinus bursa area.

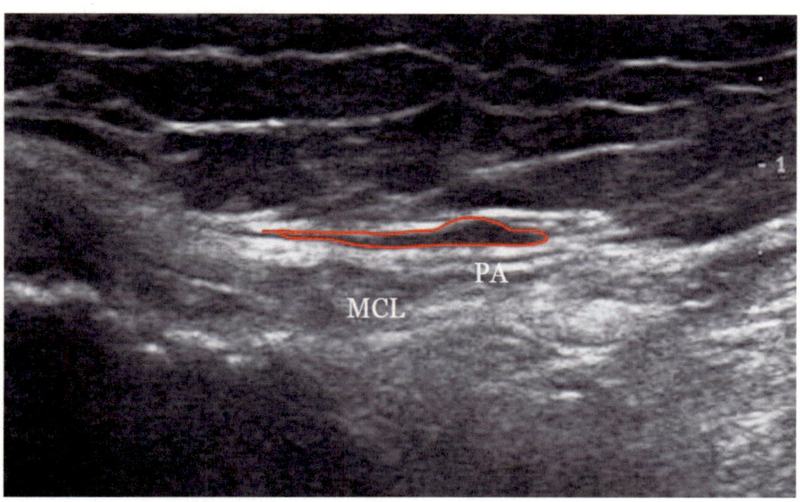

Figure 5.
Ultrasound image of the injectate location after injection; extra-pes anserinus bursa area, the injection was superficial to the tendon.

5. Discussion

The US is widely used for diagnosis and treatment in musculoskeletal fields. There have been several studies representing US features of PA tendon or PAB in patients with PATB. Some studies reported that the US is limited in detecting PATB, while others concluded that it can be helpful. Uson et al. [17] assessed the US findings of the PA and the subcutaneous fat of medial knee in clinically diagnosed PATB patients. The diagnostic findings were the thickness of the insertion of the tendons, the presence of fluid collection greater than 2 mm in the bursa, and changes in the subcutaneous fat of the medial aspect of the knee. For a total of 37 participants, PA tendinitis was diagnosed in just one knee and PA bursitis in three knees (two symptomatic and one asymptomatic). From the results, they concluded that it was difficult to detect US findings of PA tendinitis or bursitis in patients diagnosed with PATB syndrome. Unlu et al. [18] examined US evidence of PA tendinitis or bursitis in patients with type 2 diabetes mellitus. Only 8.3% of 48 patients were found to have PA tendinitis findings in the US. Although PA tendinitis or bursitis syndrome is not uncommon in patients with diabetes mellitus, there might be less frequent morphologic US changes of the PA tendons. Yoon et al. [2] prospectively studied the correlation between US findings and response to steroid injection in 26 patients with clinically diagnosed PATB syndrome. Only two patients (8.7%) showed sonographic evidence of PATB. One patient with PA tendinitis showed thickening and loss of normal fibrillar echotexture. The other who had bursitis revealed circumscribed anechoic fluid collection of 2 mm or greater.

Uysal et al. [12] evaluated the prevalence of PA bursitis in OA patients. A total of 170 knees from 85 patients with knee OA were assessed, and 20% (34/170) of the knees showed PA bursitis in US examinations. They suggested that PA bursitis was easily found in the US, and there was a positive correlation between OA grade and PAB size and area. Toktas et al. [19] studied the US findings of PA tendon and bursa in 183 clinically diagnosed PATB among the 314 knees with OA. The results showed that the mean thickness of PA in knees with OA with/without PATB was significantly greater than the controls. US could be a useful diagnostic tool for detecting PATB syndrome in knee OA patients.

The term PATB is generally used to describe the inflammatory condition of PAB; however, the structure associated with symptoms is still not identified. After the intervention in our study, all injectates (25 of 25 subjects) were located accurately in the PAB in the US-guided injection group, whereas just 18% (4 of 22 subjects) were properly located in the blind injection group. The US-guided group revealed greater pain reduction significantly than the blind group. This suggests that the pain might be arisen from the bursa, so a diagnosis of tendinobursitis is more suitable for this condition.

As previous studies have shown, US-guided injections are more accurate than blind injections. Various reviews have recently been reported on the clinical utility of US-guided injections in locations such as shoulder girdles, hip joints, and knee joints. A systematic review of US-guided shoulder girdle injections reviewed four cadaveric studies and nine human studies, and concluded that US-guided injections had greater accuracy for all types of shoulder injections than landmark-guided injections, except subacromial injection. The efficacy for the subacromial and biceps tendon sheath injections was improved [20]. Another systematic review of US-guided hip joint injections showed the improvement of accuracy. They reviewed four US-guided and five landmark-guided studies, and suggested that US-guided hip injections were significantly more accurate than landmark-guided techniques [21].

A review of US-guided intra-articular knee injections revealed that US-guided injections notably improved accuracy in the intra-articular joint injections than conventional palpation-guided injections by analyzing a total of 13 previous studies. US guidance also directly improved patient-reported clinical outcomes and cost-effectiveness [15].

PAB injection is usually performed by blind technique in actual clinical settings because PA is located closer to the superficial layer compared to other deep joints. Acromioclavicular joint (AC) is also located superficially, and blind injection is often performed through palpation. Nevertheless, a previous study has shown that the use of US in the AC joint injection is more accurate and effective [22]. They concluded that US-guided AC joint articular injection resulted in better pain and functional status improvement than palpation-guided injection at the 6-month follow-up. Therefore, even in the superficial structures, US-guided injection is recommended for accurate treatment.

For this reason, although the effectiveness of US examination in the PATB diagnosis is controversial, the value of US-guided injection treatment is sufficiently recognized for its accuracy. Overall, the accuracy of blind injections is 40–80%, while that of US-guided injections is approximately 90–100%. In most of these injections, the improved accuracy achieved by US guidance directly enhances clinical outcomes.

Consistent with previous studies, this research observed that US-guided injection was more accurate than the blind injection, and intra-bursal injection had a better clinical result in the treatment of PATB. Although the standardized US-guided injection technique has not yet been established, longitudinal access to the tibia would be appropriate to administer materials. Anatomically, the transducer is positioned in a longitudinal orientation relative to the MCL, oblique transverse access relative to the PA. While monitoring the image, insert the needle through the skin proximal to the transducer and advance in a proximal to the distal direction in a longitudinal plane. According to the physician's preference, a needle can approach the distal to the transducer and advance in the proximal direction in a longitudinal plane. The target of the injection is the space beneath the PA tendon. When the needle tip is visualized in the target space, inject the materials slowly and carefully, since the space is relatively narrow.

The PAB corticosteroid injections are contraindicated in patients with systemic infection states (sepsis, bacteremia, etc.), joint infection (septic arthritis, cellulitis, osteomyelitis, etc.), fracture, osteoporosis, coagulopathy, skin defect, hypersensitivity to the steroid, uncontrolled hyperglycemia; also, some complications such as bleeding, bruising, swelling, infection, post-injection pain (steroid flare), face flushing, skin depigmentation, cutaneous atrophy can occur [23].

There were several limitations of our study. Because of the short-term follow-up period, the long-term clinical effects could not be determined. The morphologic US features of the anserine bursa or tendon were not examined that might help to identify the source of pain in PATB. In addition, potential differences caused by activity levels were not considered even if they had a potential impact on the results of the study.

6. Conclusion

Both US-guided and blind injections significantly reduced pain levels in patients with PATB. In the US-guided injection group, the accuracy was higher than in the blind injection group. Clinical results were more affected in the US group.

All injectates were located in the PAB after the US-guided injections, while only in some cases of the blind approaches, injectates were located in the PAB. This suggests that the optimal source of pain might be associated with the bursa.

Conflict of interest

The authors declare no conflict of interest.

Author details

Jong Hwa Lee*, Jae Uk Lee and Seung Wan Yoo
Department of Physical Medicine and Rehabilitation, Dong-A University College of Medicine, Busan, Republic of Korea

*Address all correspondence to: jhlee08@dau.ac.kr

References

[1] Helfenstein M Jr, Kuromoto J. Anserine syndrome. Revista Brasileira de Reumatologia. 2010;**50**:313-327

[2] Yoon HS, Kim SE, Suh YR, Seo YI, Kim HA. Correlation between ultrasonographic findings and the response to corticosteroid injection in pes anserinus tendinobursitis syndrome in knee osteoarthritis patients. Journal of Korean Medical Science. 2005;**20**:109-112. DOI: 10.3346/jkms.2005.20.1.109

[3] Marra MD, Crema MD, Chung M, Roemer FW, Hunter DJ, Zaim S, et al. MRI features of cystic lesions around the knee. The Knee. 2008;**15**:423-438. DOI: 10.1016/j.knee.2008.04.009

[4] Handy JR. Anserine bursitis: A brief review. Southern Medical Journal. 1997;**90**:376-377. DOI: 097/00007611-199704000-00002

[5] Moschcowitz E. Bursitis of sartorius bursa, an undescribed malady simulating chronic arthritis. Journal of the American Medical Association. 1937;**109**:1362-1366. DOI: 10.1001/jama.1937.92780430001009

[6] Kang I, Han SW. Anserine bursitis in patients with osteoarthritis of the knee. Southern Medical Journal. 2000;**93**: 207-209

[7] Brookler MI, Mongan ES. Anserine bursitis, a treatable cause of knee pain in patients with degenerative arthritis. California Medicine. 1973;**119**:8-10

[8] Cohen SE, Mahul O, Meir R, et al. Anserine bursitis and noninsulin dependent diabetes mellitus. The Journal of Rheumatology. 1997;**24**: 2162-2165

[9] Klippel JH. Primer on the Rheumatic Diseases. Musculoskeletal Signs and Symptoms—Regional Rheumatic Pain Syndromes— Disorders of the Knee Region. 12th ed. Arthritis Foundation, New York: Springer; 2001. p. 182. DOI: 10.1007/978-0-387-68566-3

[10] Finnoff JT, Nutz DJ, Henning PT, Hollman JH, Smith j. Accuracy of ultrasound-guided versus unguided pes anserinus bursa injections. PM & R: The Journal of Injury, Function, and Rehabilitation. 2010;**2**:732-739. DOI: 10.1016/j.pmrj.2010.03.014

[11] Rennie WJ, Saifuddin A. Pes anserine bursitis: Incidence in symptomatic knees and clinical presentation. Skeletal Radiology. 2005;**34**:395-398. DOI: 10.1007/s00256-005-0918-7

[12] Uysal F, Akbal A, Gökmen F, Adam G, Reşorlu M. Prevalence of pes anserine bursitis in symptomatic osteoarthritis patients: An ultrasonographic prospective study. Clinical Rheumatology. 2015;**34**:529-533. DOI: 10.1007/s10067-014-2653-8

[13] Koh WL, Kwek JW, Quek ST, Peh WCG. Clinics in diagnostic imaging. Singapore Medical Journal. 2002;**43**: 485-491

[14] Gilliland CA, Salazar LD, Borchers JR. Ultrasound versus anatomic guidance for intra-articular and periarticular injection: A systematic review. The Physician and Sportsmedicine. 2011;**39**:121-131. DOI: 10.3810/psm.2011.09.1928

[15] Berkoff DJ, Miller LE, Block JE. Clinical utility of ultrasound guidance for intra-articular knee injections: A review. Clinical Interventions in Aging. 2012;**7**:89-95. DOI: 10.2147/CIA.S29265

[16] Brock G, Gurekas V. The occasional pes anserinus bursitis injection. Canadian Journal of Rural Medicine. 2014;**19**:71-73

[17] Uson J, Aguado P, Bernad M, Mayordomo L, Naredo E, Balsa A, et al. Pes anserinus tendino-bursitis: What are we talking about? Scandinavian Journal of Rheumatology. 2000;**29**:184-186. DOI: 10.1080/030097400750002076

[18] Unlu Z, Ozmen B, Tarhan S, Boyvoda S, Goktan C. Ultrasonographic evaluation of pes anserinus tendino-bursitis in patients with type 2 diabetes mellitus. The Journal of Rheumatology. 2003;**30**:352-354

[19] Toktas H, Dundar U, Adar S, Solak O, Ulasil AM. Ultrasonographic assessment of pes anserinus tendon and pes anserinus tendinitis bursitis syndrome in patients with knee osteoarthritis. Modern Rheumatology. 2015;**25**:128-133. DOI: 10.3109/14397595.2014.931909

[20] Aly AR, Rajasekaran S, Ashworth N. Ultrasound-guided shoulder girdle injections are more accurate and more effective than landmark-guided injections: A systematic review and meta-analysis. British Journal of Sports Medicine. 2015;**49**:1042-1049. DOI: 10.1136/bjsports-2014-093573

[21] Hoeber S, Aly AR, Ashworth N, Rajasekaran S. Ultrasound-guided hip joint injections are more accurate than landmark-guided injections: A systematic review and meta-analysis. British Journal of Sports Medicine. 2016;**50**:392-396. DOI: 10.1136/bjsports-2014-094570

[22] Park KD, Kim TK, Lee J, Lee WY, Ahn JK, Park Y. Palpation versus ultrasound-guided acromioclavicular joint intra-articular corticosteroid injections: A retrospective comparative clinical study. Pain Physician. 2015;**18**:333-341

[23] Simurina T, Mraovic B, Zupcic M, Zupcic SG, Vulin M. Local anesthetics and steroids: Contraindications and complications-clinical update. Acta Clinica Croatica. 2019;**58**:53-61

Chapter 8

Revision of Training Models on Ultrasound-Guided Vascular Access: Presentation of an Animal Model

J.M. López Álvarez, O. Pérez Quevedo, S. Alonso-Graña López-Manteola, J. Naya Esteban, J.F. Loro Ferrer and D.L. Lorenzo Villegas

Abstract

Simulation has been defined as the representation of something as real. It is necessary for performing the ultrasound-guided vascular cannulation technique correctly. The use of training models for diagnostic or therapeutic procedures: improves the quality of care for patients; decreases stress level that it can produce the realization of a new technique directly on the patient and; can be used as many times as the model is reproduced, also serving as a method for the resolution of some problems that may appear related to the in vivo technique. The evidence shows that simulation plays an important role in the acquisition of skills to perform invasive procedures. The use of ultrasound in vascular accesses whether peripheral or central, arterial, or venous, improves the success rate in the canalization and reduce the complications derived from the technique in certain critical situations (coagulopathy, thrombocytopenia, obesity, etc.) specially in pediatric patients given the variability of depth and diameter of its vessels with respect to the adult population. To facilitate learning in the technique of echoguided puncture, a training model is presented that is easily reproducible, economical and with a high fidelity in relation to the punctures performed on the patient.

Keywords: training, simulation, model, ultrasound

1. Introduction

Simulation has been defined as the presentation of something as real, it means a situation in which some conditions are artificially created to resemble the reality [1–3]. This is used with the objectives of studying something or training in a new medical procedure. To implement a technique such as the ultrasound-guided vascular access, a series of skills must be acquired in order to reach the required aptitudes to perform vascular cannulations in a proper manner [2–5].

These skills include the following: (a) knowledge and comprehension of the device to be used as well as their technical bases, in our study, the ultrasound machine and ultrasonography; (b) the visualization and optimization of the vascular image and of the needle, and; (c) the ability to acquire the required skills to use the ultrasound probe and to insert the needle (puncture) when performing the procedure of ultrasound-guided vascular access [6–11].

The use of simulation models as diagnostic or therapeutic procedures training models has the following advantages: (a) they increase patients' assistance quality, especially if these techniques are associated to complications and risks; (b) they decrease the stress level eventually provoked by the direct performance of a new technique on patients, and; (c) they can be used as many times as the model is reproduced, so they can be additionally used to solve some problems that could arise from the "in vivo" performance of the technique [10, 12, 13].

Evidence shows that simulation plays an important role in the acquisition of skills required to perform invasive procedures [13, 14]. The use of ultrasound scan on vascular access increases the success rate of the cannulation and reduce the complications derived from this technique. Irrespective of these vessels are peripheral or central and arteries or veins [15–18]. However, the ultrasound-guided vascular access is displaced for the benefit of the classical technique ("blindly" oriented by anatomic references) by some reasons, such as the learning curve that every invasive technique requires and the ultrasound machine preparation required to perform this technique (probe sterilization, choice of the proper "pre-set," puncture plane, etc.). The preference for the classical technique occurs even when it takes the risk of complications associated, which increase under certain critical conditions (coagulopathy, thrombocytopenia, obesity, etc.). These considerations are especially relevant in pediatric patients due to their vessels' depth and diameter variability, which is higher than in adult patients [19, 20].

2. Model types

It is noticeable that experimental, simulation, or no-human models are used infrequently in learning invasive techniques/procedures such as ultrasound-guided vascular access. Any training process on a simulation model represents an opportunity to practice the technique without taking risks and entails the learning of the use of ultrasounds. All of the above is feasible to increase patients' security when performing invasive procedures on children [8, 13].

The training models usually are extremely expensive, hardly available, or not good at transmitting ultrasounds in an optimal manner.

Most of the training or experimental models than can be used to perform simulations for the ultrasound-guided vascular access training are synthetic or biological. Some of them are commercially available and other can be constructed manually by any person [11, 21–23]. They are the following: (a) "in vivo" models performed on research animals; (b) commercially available models such as Blue Phantom® or silicon or latex models, and; (c) synthetic handcrafted models constructed by using gelatine/agar or tissue animal models constructed by using chicken thighs, turkey thighs, or chicken breast [14, 24, 25]. Each of these models must contains tubular structures inside, that can be made on plastic, latex, or rubber, and filled with liquid, in order to simulate the vessels to be cannulated.

These models can be classified as cannulation-puncture models or puncture-localization models depending on the use of them.

2.1 Characteristics of an ideal training model

An ideal training model to perform ultrasound-guided vascular access procedures should:

- reproduce texture and resistance of human tissue;
- have enough penetration surface to transmit correctly the ultrasounds;
- permit the identification and localization of the different tissue structures;
- obtain an optimal image;
- permit different difficulty and complexity levels when the procedure is performed;
- avoid, to the extent possible, the visibility of the puncture needle path;
- permit the visualization of the needle;
- have long average life;
- be easily transportable, and reproducible in any environment;
- be easily available and inexpensive.

3. Advantages and disadvantages of the different ultrasound-guided vascular access training models

3.1 Blue Phantom®

Commercially available simulator to be used as a training model of procedures in which ultrasounds are used as vascular access guides (**Figure 1**).

They are expensive, not-transportable, and not-changeable, although the latest models permit even simulate arterial pulse (**Figure 2**). The puncture needle entry point and path usually remain visible. The puncture performance sensation on this model is different from that on human tissues. They require maintenance and deteriorates after multiple puncture performances. They are not easily available nor affordable [21–23].

3.2 Silicone models

Commercially available models consisting of a silicone model containing a tubular structure which permits the vascular access simulation and that can be refilled after each puncture performance. They have a long average life, and they are easily transportable. However, they offer a small surface area due to their small size, they are expensive and not easily available to all [11, 26, 27]. The puncture needle entry point and path remain visible after multiple puncture performances (**Figure 3**).

3.3 Agar/gelatine models

It consists of an agar or gelatine model in which a tubular elastic structure is inserted (in some cases, Penrose surgical drains of different sizes). They have been used by radiologists to train and teach ultrasound-guided procedures (**Figure 4**). They are easy to construct by using everyday kitchen utensils and they are ideal for hand-eye coordination learning and improvement [28, 29].

However: (a) they usually show an uniform appearance of the ultrasound image (**Figure 5**) without identifiable muscle or tendon structures (with the exception of preparations including any component like mucilage); (b) the puncture needle

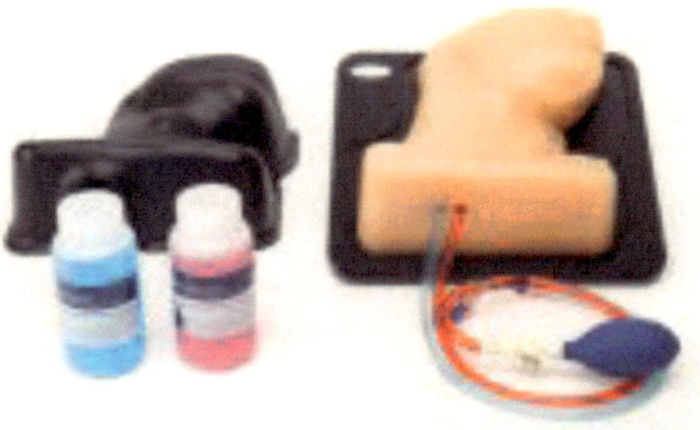

Figure 1.
Blue Phantom® model.

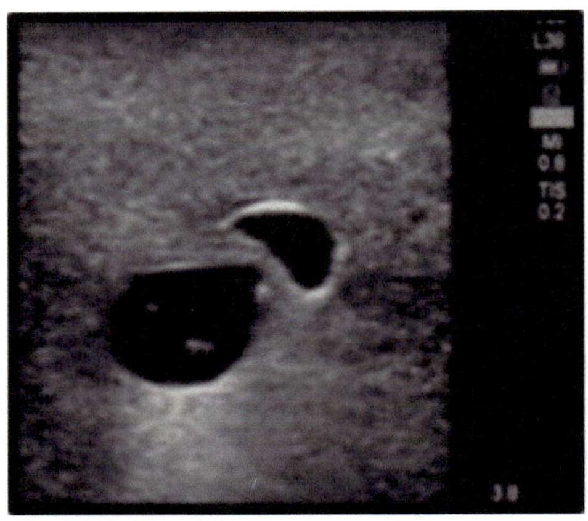

Figure 2.
Ultrasound image of internal jugular vein and carotid artery (Blue Phantom® model).

entry point and path remain visible after some puncture performances; (c) their puncture performance sensation is different from that on human tissues; (d) depending on the gelatine concentration used during their construction, they can be easily damaged, and; (e) the needle sideways movements during its introduction into the agar/gelatine could be hardly controllable when trying to puncture the vessel.

3.4 Animal models

(a) "In vivo": the use of research animals results in high cost and laborious preparation when optimal conditions are required (sedation, mechanical ventilation or respiratory support, monitoring, etc.) as well as in a limited number of punctures; (b) "artificial": they are manually constructed by using pork, turkey or chicken thighs, pork-belly, tofu or sausage/cold meat piece as *muscle structure*, and different elastic components (urinary catheters, chest drains, metallic trocar, serum infusion systems, etc.) as *vascular structure*. By using them, a real sensation

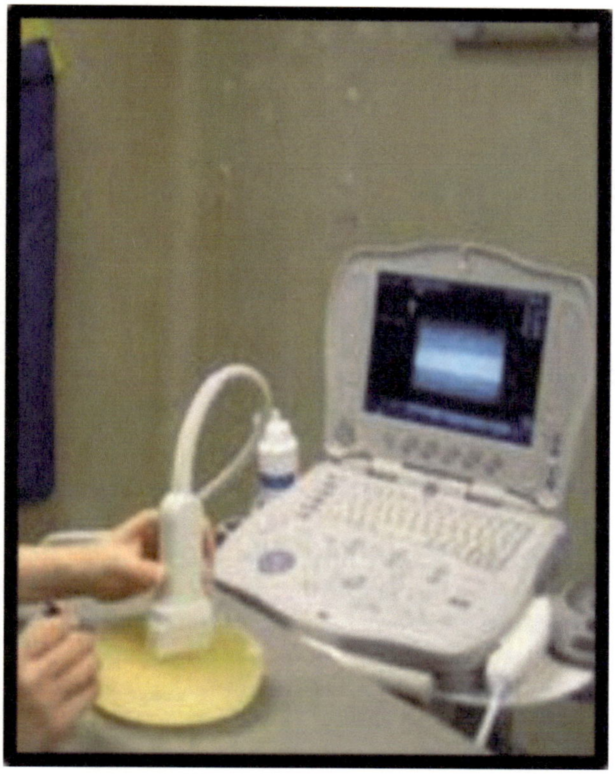

Figure 3.
Silicone model for ultrasound-guided vascular access.

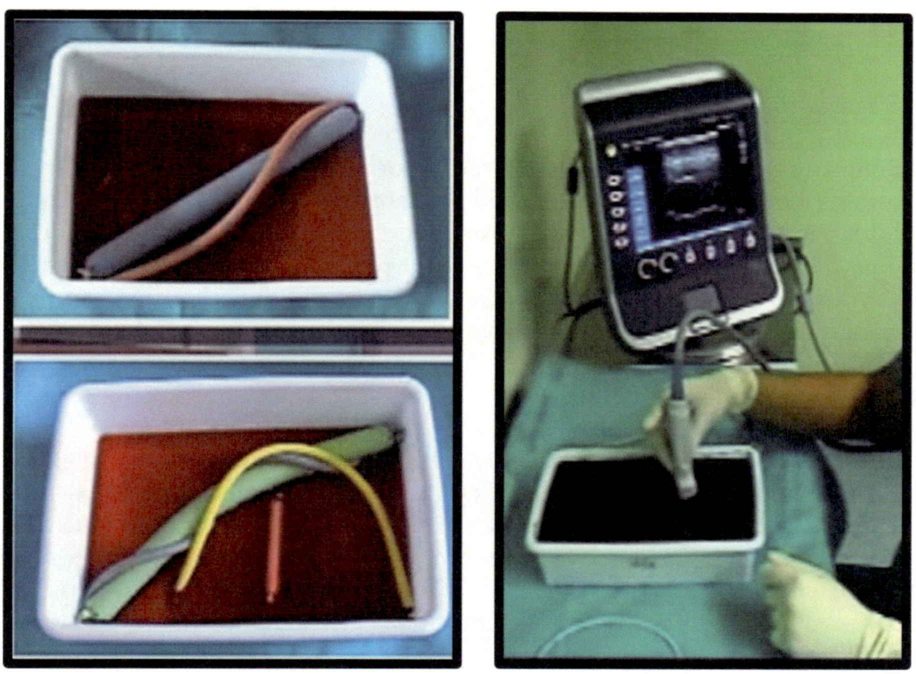

Figure 4.
Gelatine model: Penrose drains using different water-soluble colorants, which are fixed to different gelatine layers (image courtesy of Dr. Vicente Roqués).

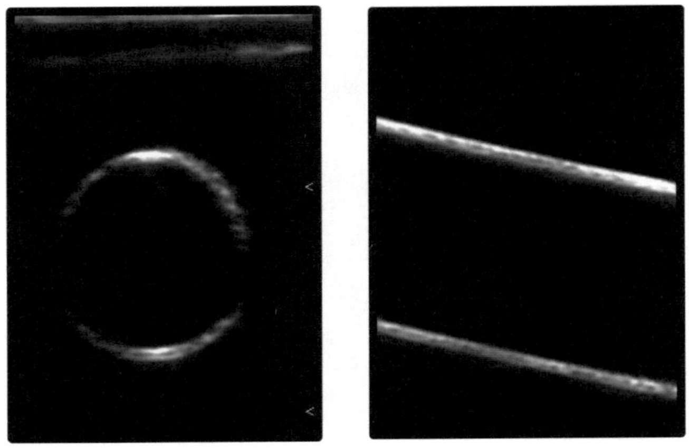

Figure 5.
Ultrasound image of transversal axis (left) and longitudinal axis (right) within the gelatine model.

of different tissues is created with respect to both the ultrasound image perspective and the sensation obtained when performing puncture and cannulation/vascular access. These models show an affordable preparation, but their construction needs a certain amount of time. In addition, they are inexpensive as well as easily transportable and manageable. Their design permits different complexity levels with respect to different vessels diameter and depth, so the difficulty level can be increased as progress is made on the training process. With respect to their disadvantages, these models' conservation needs refrigeration, their average life is short (some weeks to get their muscle structure deteriorated) and they must be carefully constructed in order to reduce their risk of air introduction into their vascular structure [8, 15, 25].

The main advantages and disadvantages of the main cannulation-puncture models are shown in **Table 1**.

3.5 Simulation software

Simulators provided with high software-algorithm-based fidelity have been used as training models on ultrasound-guided procedures. Their disadvantages include their high cost and the need for software support. Their advantages include the absolute lack of infection control problems, the possibility of changing the complexity/difficulty level. Simulators can be installed in not clinical settings, such as training rooms, and they can be available at any time of the day or night [30, 31].

3.6 Puncture-localization models

These are artificial models frequently used by radiologists for the training on localization and puncture of nodular or cystic structures, mainly hepatic mammary or thyroid ones [11, 26, 27]. These models are used to get familiarize with the ultrasound machine and with the puncture technique in ultrasound-guided procedures. The *tissue/muscle component* can be: piece of poultry breast, liver or tofu, sausage/cold meat piece or surgical gloves filled with a warm water dilution containing food thickener. The *vascular/nodular component* can be whole/pitted olives, cheese puffs-blocks, jelly beans or gumdrops, wires or knitting needles, etc. and they must be included inside the tissue/muscle component (**Figure 6**).

Models	Advantages	Disadvantages
Blue Phantom®	Transportable	Human tissue texture not reproduced
	Long average life	Very visible puncture needle entry point
	Large surface area	Poor resemblance to real vascular and muscular images
		Expensive
Silicone	Transportable	Small surface area
	Long average life	Expensive
		Very visible puncture needle path
Agar/gelatine	Transportable	Uniform appearance of ultrasound image
	Inexpensive	Human tissue texture not reproduced
	Easy construction	Strong puncture needle path
		Easily damaged
		Possible air artifacts within the vascular structure
Animal "in vivo"	High resemblance to reality	Not transportable
	Large surface area	Expensive
		Large facility and authorization required
		Limited needle punctures
Animal "artificial"	Transportable	Short average life
	Easy construction	Preparation time required
	Inexpensive	Possible air artifacts within the vascular structure
	Human tissue texture reproduced	
	High resemblance to real vascular and muscular images	

Table 1.
Training models for ultrasound-guided vascular access: "pros and cons."

4. Animal model construction and description

The training model described here consists of the following [8]:

4.1 Muscle component

Piece of bird breast that can be acquired at any grocery store/shop and with the following approximated measures (length, width, height): 10 cm × 10 cm × 3 cm (**Figure 7**). Frozen poultry breast is preferably used; being defrosted in a refrigerator within 24 hours before performing the vascular punctures.

4.2 Vascular component

Tubular structure made in elastic material (modeling balloon) filled with 10 ml of water with water-soluble colorant and sealed on both sides by using knots (**Figure 8**).

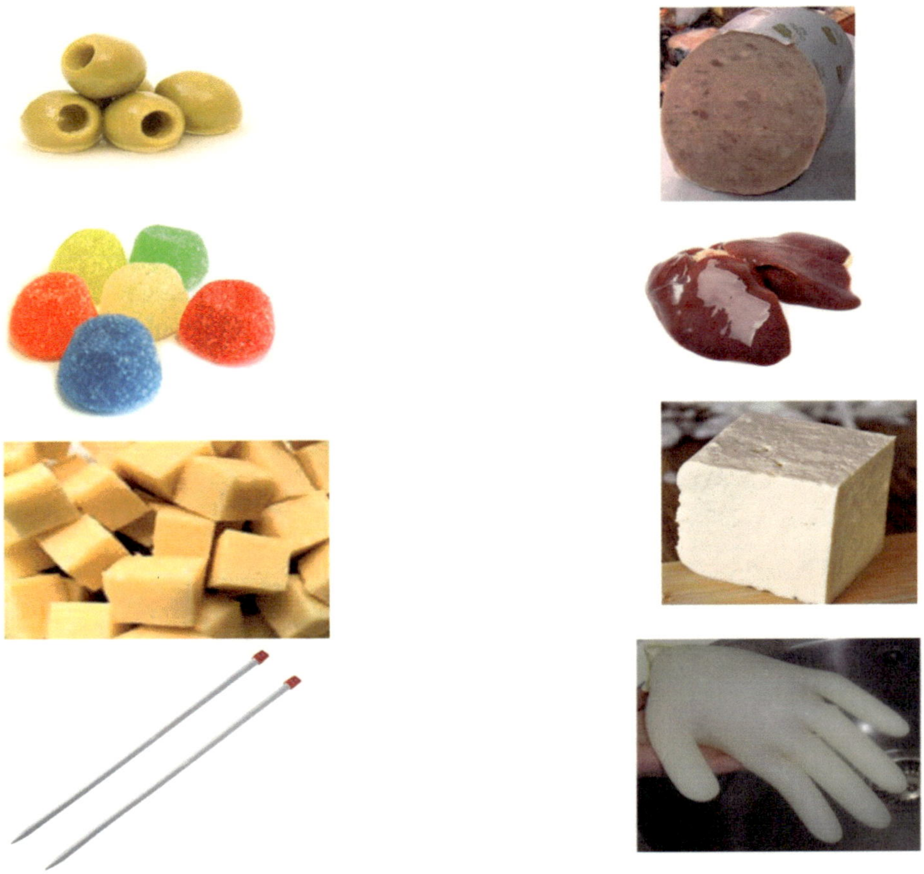

Figure 6.
Components of different puncture-localization models. Left: vascular-nodular structure. Right: tissue-muscle structure.

Both components simulate the muscle and the vascular structures of pediatric patients. The development of this model is based on the introduction of an eight French thoracic drain together with its puncture trocar passing longitudinally through the muscle component and at different depth levels. This simulates the different depths at which vessels are located in children depending on their age and weight. After that, the trocar is retired, and the drain plastic piece remains inside the muscle structure. In the drain distal part, the elastic tubular structure distal end is sutured in the knot area. When pulling the drain in the opposite direction, the device stays inside the muscle structure and then, it is prepared to be visualized and cannulated in an ultrasound-guided manner in this experimental model (**Figure 9**).

A system of clamps fixed at different length permits the application of different tension values on the elastic structure. Depending on these different tension values, three different diameter ranges can be obtained, which are comparable to pediatric patients' vessels diameters. Thus, different ultrasound-guided vascular access difficulty levels can be obtained (**Figure 10**).

To perform puncture and cannulation, a 3-French and 11-cm-length catheter is used, with a 30-cm radiopaque guide and a 5.5-mm needle. Each unit of this model permits the performance of more than 100 punctures without resulting

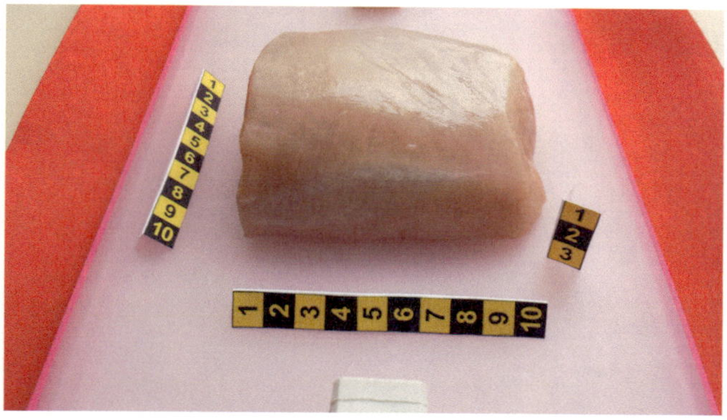

Figure 7.
Training model muscle component sizes.

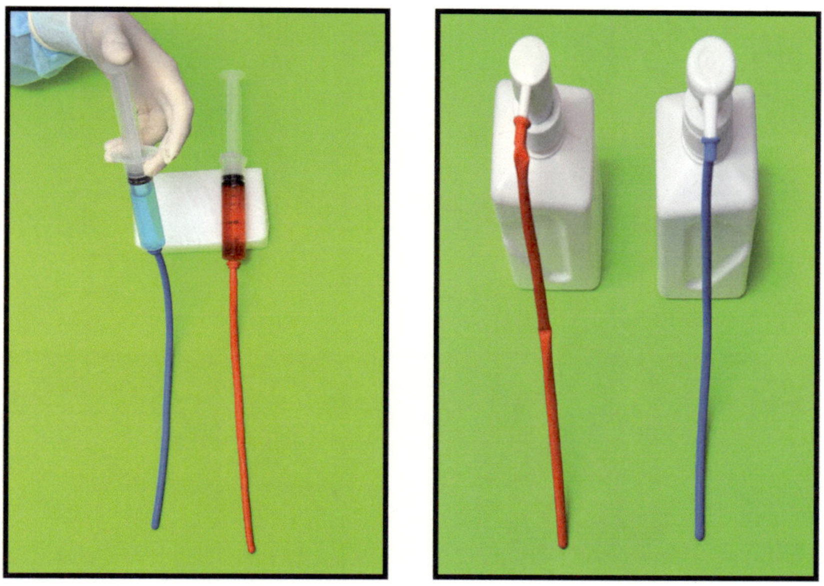

Figure 8.
Vascular structure filling with water-soluble colorant, by using a syringe (left) or a dispenser (right).

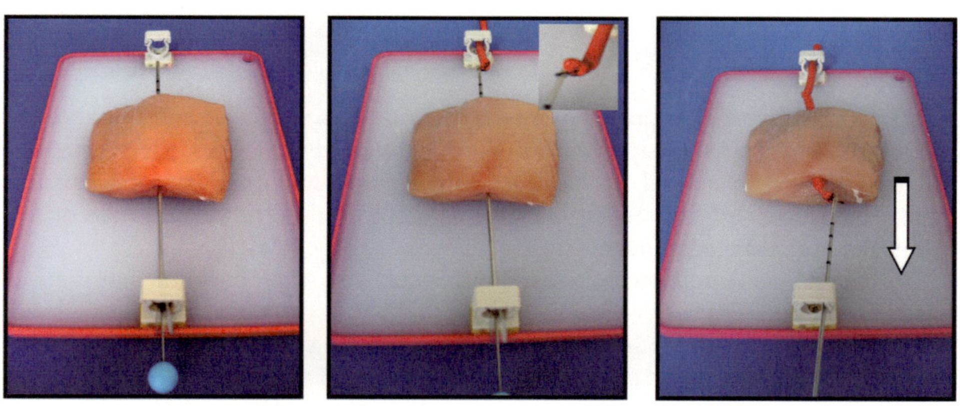

Figure 9.
Left: Puncture trocar passing longitudinally through the model muscle tissue. Middle: Drain suture on the side of the vascular structure which is isolated distal portion (details in the upper-right corner). Right: Placement of the vascular structure inside the muscle structure, and after the traction of the drain sutured to the vascular structure.

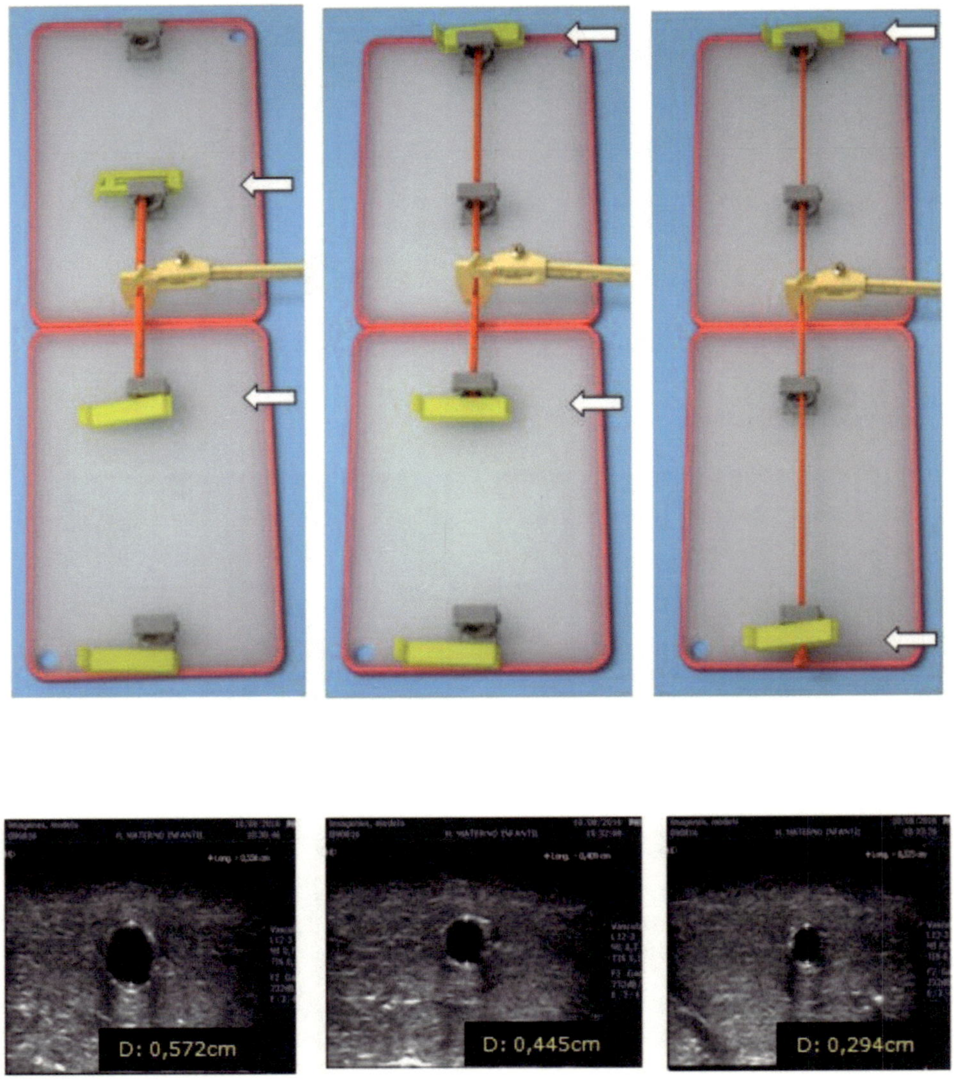

Figure 10.
Vessel's diameters (D1–D3) depending on the stretching degree of the elastic structure with its clamps (arrows) and their ultrasound representation.

deteriorated at a cost of approximately 3 €. The model is replicable and reusable, and it lasts for approximately 6 hours at room temperature. When sessions last less than 6 hours, the model can be stored in an airtight container and refrigerated again. This increases its durability without affecting neither the visualization quality nor the puncture technique.

Ultrasound gel or aqueous solution (double-distilled water or saline 0.9%) are recommended to get a better visualization of the vascular structures.

By using a linear probe ultrasound machine, choosing the "preset vascular," and 2-cm depth, the vascular structure in the training model as well as its correlation with the real image "in vivo" in the patient can be observed (**Figure 11**).

After visualizing the vessel, the depth and diameter of the elastic tubular structure, which is similar to the pediatric patient's vessel, are determined.

It can be stablished 3 depth levels and 3 diameter levels according to preliminary results from 300 depth and diameter measurements of the most common pediatric patients' central vessels. Within these data, different weights and sizes referenced by our group were found (**Table 2**). These measurements were valid with a 99% reliability.

The average values of these measurements are included within nine categories obtained by combining different vessels depths (three ranges) and diameters (three ranges) inside the muscular structure of the training model (**Table 3**).

The training model described permits to perform vessel puncture and cannulation in an ultrasound-guided manner in the three most used vascular-access ultrasound axes: transverse axis-out of plane, oblique axis-in plane, and longitudinal axis-in plane (**Figures 12–14**).

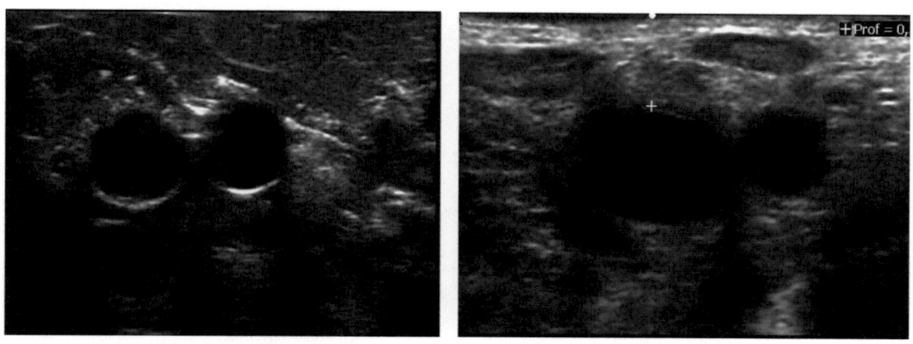

Figure 11.
Experimental training model image (left) with respect to the "in vivo" real image (right).

Weight range	Depth average (SD)	Diameter average (SD)
<10 kg	0.56 cm (0.14)	0.30 cm (0.03)
10–30 kg	0.65 cm (0.17)	0.50 cm (0.18)
30–50 kg	0.90 cm (0.24)	0.69 cm (0.08)
>50 kg	1.65 cm (0.14)	0.70 cm (0.03)

SD, standard deviation.

Table 2.
Depth and diameter measurements (in centimeters: cm) of the main central vessels within the pediatric population (n = 300).

Depth	Diameter
P1: 0.5–1.0 cm	D1: 0.51–0.65 cm
P2: 1.01–1.50 cm	D2: 0.36–0.50 cm
P3: 1.51–2.0 cm	D3: 0.20–0.35 cm

Table 3.
Depth ranges (P1–3) and diameter ranges (D1–3) measured in centimeters (cm) used in the training model for ultrasound-guided vascular access.

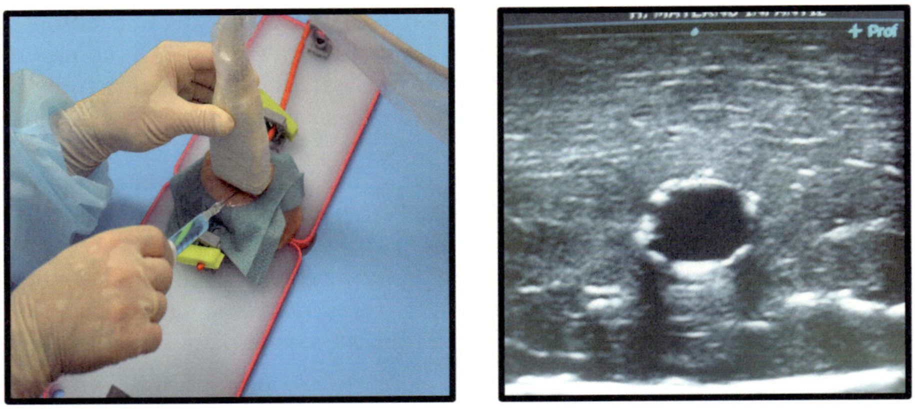

Figure 12.
Left: Puncture needle in the transverse axis-out of plane. Right: Vascular structure ultrasound image in the transverse axis-out of plane.

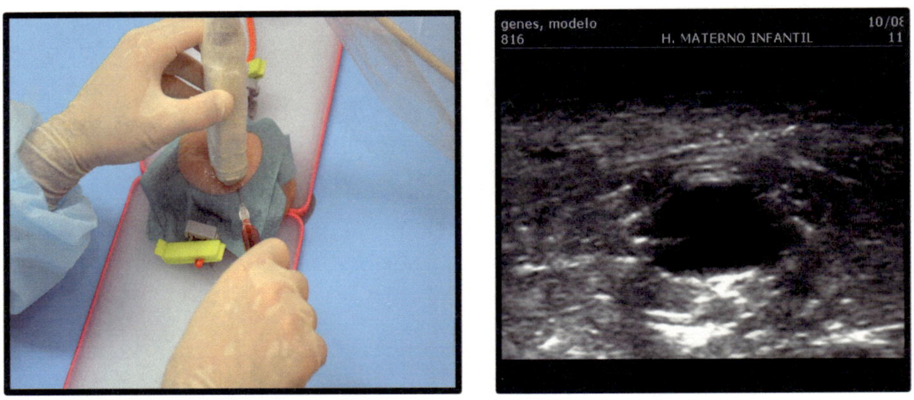

Figure 13.
Vascular visualization and image of the puncture needle in the oblique axis-in plane.

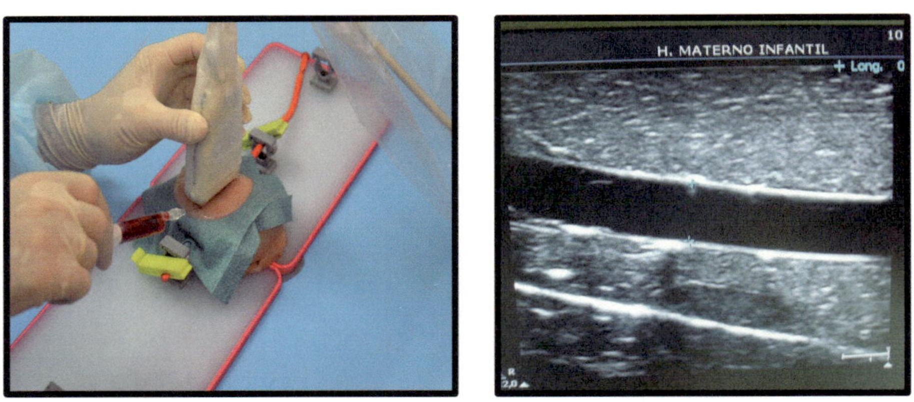

Figure 14.
Vascular visualization and image of the puncture needle in the longitudinal axis-in plane.

5. Considerations to be highlighted with respect to the training models on ultrasound-guided vascular access

Ultrasound-guided vascular access is a tool to decrease the probability of making errors, the risk of complications, and the number of attempts when performing a vascular access [10, 12, 13, 32].

This technique requires a proper training in order to optimize the learning curve which is characteristic of every invasive procedure [17, 18].

Every simulation model, even the most rudimentary and crude, is a useful tool to improve the results of ultrasound-guided vascular access. It will make it possible to minimize the probability of complications and, with respect to the professionals performing this technique, their trust in this technique performance will be increased [11, 14, 24].

The simulation model described by our research team to perform ultrasound-guided vascular access has been used in more than 800 punctures [8, 17, 18]. After testing most of the previously described models, it could be said that the structure provided by this model is closely similar to pediatric patient's muscular and vascular structures, and that it resembles these patients' vessels anatomy, depth, and diameter with respect to the children's weight. This model improves the learning curve to acquire the skill required by this technique when it is performed by doctors trained in vascular access by following the instructions of the classical technique ("blindly" oriented by anatomic references), by doctors not trained in vascular access or by nurses to cannulate peripherally inserted central catheter [14, 24].

This model is inexpensive, easy to prepare and transportable, and it permits the visualization of the vascular structures, the measurement of these structures, the ultrasound-guided cannulation, and the visualization of the needle from the different ultrasound axes. It also permits maneuvering in response to access difficulties, such as needle replacement/reinsertion, and checking the correct cannulation by visualizing the guide inside the vascular structure [8].

In addition, this model reproduces the different depth and diameter ranges of children's vessels. So, taken together with the above, each simulation performed by using this model can be used to develop the skills required to perform ultrasound-guided vascular accesses [19, 20].

Author details

J.M. López Álvarez[1,2*], O. Pérez Quevedo[1], S. Alonso-Graña López-Manteola[1], J. Naya Esteban[2,3], J.F. Loro Ferrer[4] and D.L. Lorenzo Villegas[5]

1 Unit of Pediatric Intensive Medicine, Mother and Child University Hospital of the Canary Islands, Canary Islands, Spain

2 Department of Nursing, Fernando Pessoa-Canarias University, Las Palmas de Gran Canaria, Spain

3 Unit of Interventive Vascular Radiology, Mother and Child University Hospital of the Canary Islands, Canary Islands, Spain

4 Department of Clinical Sciences, University of Las Palmas de Gran Canaria, Spain

5 Fernando Pessoa-Canarias University, Las Palmas, Spain

*Address all correspondence to: jmloal@hotmail.com

References

[1] Nestel D, Groom J, Eikeland-Husebø S, O'Donnell JM. Simulation for learning and teaching procedural skills: The state of the science. Simulation in Healthcare. 2011;**Suppl.6**(7):S10-S13. DOI: 10.1097/SIH.0b013e318227ce96

[2] Schmidt GA, Kory P. Ultrasound-guided central venous catheter insertion: Teaching and learning. Intensive Care Medicine. 2014;**40**:111-113

[3] Rothschild JM. Ultrasound guidance of central vein catheterization. In: Making Health Care Safer: A Critical Analysis of Patient Safety Practices. Evidence Report/Technology Assessment: Number 43. AHRQ Publication No. 1-E058, July 2001: Chapter 21. Rockville, MD: Agency for Healthcare Research and Quality; 2001

[4] Franco Sadud R, Schnobrich D, Mathews BK, Candotti C, Abdel-Ghani S, Pérez MG, Chu Rodgers S, Mader MJ, Haro EK, Dancel R, Cho J, Grikis L, Lucas BP. Recommendations on the Use of Ultrasound Guidance for Central and Peripheral Vascular Access in Adults: A Position Statement of the Society of Hospital Medicine. 2019. Available from: https://n9.cl/p5rui

[5] Naur TMH, Nilsson PM, Pietersen PI, Clementsen PF, Konge L. Simulation-Based Training in Flexible Bronchoscopy and Endobronchial Ultrasound-Guided Transbronchial Needle Aspiration: A Systematic Review. 2017. Available from: https://n9.cl/2394

[6] Ault MJ, Rosen BT, Ault B. The use of tissue models for vascular access training. Journal of General Internal Medicine. 2006;**21**:514-517

[7] Kendall JL, Faragher JP. Ultrasound-guided central venous access: A homemade phantom for simulation. CJEM. 2007;**9**:371-373

[8] Pérez Quevedo O, López Alvarez JM, Limiñana Cañal JM, Loro Ferrer JF. Design and application of model for training ultrasound-guided vascular cannulation in pediatric patients. Medicina Intensiva. 2016;**40**(6):364-370. DOI: 10.1016/j.medin.2015.11.005

[9] Rippey JCR, Blanco P, Carr PJ. An affordable easily constructed model for training in ultrasound-guided vascular access. The Journal of Vascular Access. 2015;**16**(5):422-427

[10] Moureau N et al. Evidence-based consensus on the insertion of central venous access devices: Definition of minimal requirements for training. British Journal of Anaesthesia. 2013;**110**: 347-356

[11] Kim YH. Ultrasound phantoms to protect patients from novices. The Korean Journal of Pain. 2016;**29**(2): 73-77. DOI: 10.3344/kjp.2016.29.2.73

[12] Adhikari S, Schmier C, Marx J. Focused Simulation Training: Emergency Department Nurses' Confidence and Comfort Level in Performing Ultrasound-Guided Vascular Access. 2015. Available from: https://cutt.ly/ccgRTDz

[13] Vieira RL, Gallagher RA, Stack AM, Werner HC, Levy JA. Development and evaluation of a program for the use of ultrasound for central venous catheter placement in a Pediatric Emergency Department. Pediatric Emergency Care. 2013;**29**:1245-1248

[14] Hocking G et al. A review of the benefits and pitfalls of phantoms in ultrasound-guided regional anesthesia. Regional Anesthesia and Pain Medicine. 2011;**36**:162-170

[15] Baddoo H, Djagbletey R, Owoo C. A simple tissue model for practicing ultrasound guided vascular cannulation. Ghana Medical Journal. 2014;**48**:47-49

[16] Syed Farjad S et al. Simulators for training in ultrasound guided procedures. Medical Ultrasound. 2013;**15**(2):125-131

[17] López-Álvarez JM, Pérez-Quevedo O, Naya-Esteban J, Ramirez-Lorenzo T, López-Manteola SA, Lorenzo-Villegas DL. Evaluation of training in pediatric ultrasound-guided vascular cannulation using a model. Journal of Medical Ultrasound. 2020;**29**(3):171-175. DOI: 10.4103/JMU.JMU_109_20

[18] López-Álvarez JM, Pérez-Quevedo O, Naya-Esteban J, et al. Ultrasound-guided pediatric vascular cannulation by inexperienced operators: Outcomes in a training model. Journal of Ultrasound; 2021. DOI: 10.1007/s40477-021-00585-9

[19] López Álvarez JM, Pérez Quevedo O, Santana Cabrera L, Escot CR, Loro Ferrer JF, Lorenzo TR, et al. Vascular ultrasound in pediatrics: Estimation of depth and diameter of jugular and femoral vessels. Journal of Ultrasound. 2017;**20**(4):285-292. DOI: 10.1007/s40477-017-0272-3

[20] López Alvarez JM, Pérez Quevedo O, Santana Cabrera L, Rodríguez Escot C, Ramírez Lorenzo T, Limiñana Cañal JM, et al. Vascular ultrasound in pediatrics: Utility and application of location and measurement of jugular and femoral vessels. Journal of Medical Ultrasonics. 2018;**45**(3):469-477. DOI: 10.1007/s10396-017-0853-y

[21] Schofer JM, Nomura JT, Bauman MJ, Sierzenski PR. Prospective durability testing of a vascular access phantom. The Western Journal of Emergency Medicine. 2010;**11**(4):302-305

[22] Hauglum SD, Crenshaw NA, Gattamorta KA, Mitzova-Vladinov G. Evaluation of a low-cost, high-fidelity animal model to train graduate advanced practice nursing students in the performance of ultrasound-guided central line catheter insertion. Simulation in Healthcare. 2018;**13**(5):341-347. DOI: 10.1097/SIH.0000000000000337

[23] Ryan LK, Foster FS. Tissue equivalent vessel phantoms for intravascular ultrasound. Ultrasound in Medicine & Biology. 1997;**23**(2):261-273. DOI: 10.1016/s0301-5629(96)00206-2

[24] Pepley DF, Sonntag CC, Prabhu RS, Yovanoff MA, Han DC, Miller SR, et al. Building ultrasound phantoms with modified polyvinyl chloride: A comparison of needle insertion forces and sonographic appearance with commercial and traditional simulation materials. Simulation in Healthcare. 2018;**13**(3):149-153. DOI: 10.1097/SIH.0000000000000302

[25] Sanchez-de-Toledo J, Villaverde I. Advanced low-cost ultrasound-guided vascular access simulation: The chicken breast model. Pediatric Emergency Care. 2017;**33**(9):e43-e45. DOI: 10.1097/PEC.0000000000000620

[26] Wang X, Joyce C, Kuipers JJ. Making a convenient, low-cost phantom with a previously unreported material for practicing ultrasound-guided procedures. Clinical Ultrasound. 2021;**49**(9):987-991. DOI: 10.1002/jcu.23065

[27] Kwon SY, Hong SH, Kim ES, Park HJ, You Y, Kim YH. The efficacy of lumbosacral spine phantom to improve resident proficiency in performing ultrasound-guided spinal procedure. Pain Medicine. 2015;**16**(12):2284-2291. DOI: 10.1111/pme.12870

[28] Chao SL, Chen KC, Lin LW, Wang TL, Chong CF. Ultrasound phantoms made of gelatin covered with hydrocolloid skin dressing. The Journal of Emergency Medicine. 2013;**45**(2):240-243. DOI: 10.1016/j.jemermed.2012.11.022

[29] Morrow DS, Broder J. Cost-effective, reusable, leak-resistant ultrasound-guided vascular access trainer. The Journal of Emergency Medicine. 2015;**49**(3):313-317. DOI: 10.1016/j.jemermed.2015.04.005

[30] Shanks D, Wong RY, Roberts JM, Nair P, Ma IW. Use of simulator-based medical procedural curriculum: The learner's perspectives. BMC Medical Education. 2010;**10**:77. DOI: 10.1186/1472-6920-10-77

[31] Barsuk JH, McGaghie WC, Cohen ER, O'Leary KJ, Wayne DB. Simulation-based mastery learning reduces complications during central venous catheter insertion in a medical intensive care unit. Critical Care Medicine. 2009;**37**(10):2697-2701

[32] López Álvarez JM, Pérez Quevedo O, Ramírez Lorenzo T, Limiñana Cañal JM, Loro Ferrer JF. Ultrasound-guided vascular cannulation. Experience in critically-ill pediatric patients. Archivos Argentinos de Pediatría. 2018;**116**(3):204-209. DOI: 10.5546/aap.2018.eng.204

Chapter 9

Molecular Sonography: Current and Future Applications

Arthur Fleischer and Sai Chennupati

Abstract

This communication provides an overview of the current and future applications of molecular sonography, emphasizing the principles of the technique. Molecular sonography is currently used for preclinical assessment of tumor detection and response in a variety of models. It has potential clinical applications in improved characterization of tumors based on their genomes. Clinical trials have been conducted for a variety of neoplastic, inflammatory and immunologic abnormalities.

Keywords: Labeled microbubbles, molecular characterization and detection, assessment of tumor response, ultrasonography

1. Introduction

Molecular imaging describes a relatively new imaging technique that depicts molecular processes rather than anatomic changes that occur in diseased tissue. It affords non-invasive imaging on a cellular level based on depiction of selected molecular receptors. The premise of molecular imaging is based on the fact that molecular events precede anatomic changes, and therefore, have the potential to detect neoplastic processes early as well as potentially determine response to therapy shortly after its administration. Molecular imaging can depict genomic phenotypes, and advantage that proves key to personalizing medical therapy.

There are a variety of modalities currently used to image diseased tissue. PET, or Positron Emission Tomography, utilizes radioactive substances known as tracers to detect disease. It is noninvasive and can identify areas of high metabolic activity that may be concerning for cancer. However, PET's anatomic clarity is imprecise compared to CT/MRI and it remains quite expensive. SPECT, Single Photon Emission Tomography, implements a similar mechanism as PET but is appreciably cheaper. Additionally, the radio tracers in SPECT have much longer half-lives, extending the imaging window. However, SPECT has even lower image resolution than PET. MRI, Magnetic Resonance Imaging, does not use radiation and provides a snapshot of the patient's anatomy with excellent resolution. However, it is notably time-consuming and expensive.

Molecular sonography holds many advantages over these imaging techniques. In addition to its low cost and high spatial resolution, molecular sonography is considered easy to use and repeatable when compared to most other diagnostic modalities. Currently, it is used for evaluation of tumor models. Reports of the use of molecular sonography in human subjects have recently been published [1].

This review will describe the current uses of molecular sonography and discuss future directions for research and development.

2. Targeted microbubbles

Microbubbles used for contrast enhanced and molecular sonography consist of an encapsulated gas covered by a lipid shell. They range from 2 to 5 microns in size, approximately one-third the size of an erythrocyte. As such, they remain intravascular and do not extravasate into the interstitium. They enhance the signal-to-noise ratio due to their oscillations in an insonated field as best depicted using harmonics.

A variety of targeting ligands, such as the vasogenic growth factor (VEGF) receptor, can be attached to the shell of a microbubble using the streptavidin-biotin spacer (**Figure 1**) [2]. Molecular sonography has been used to evaluate tumor angiogenesis, anti-immune encephalomyelitis, inflammatory bowel disease, transplant rejection and abnormal myocardial perfusion. The most frequently utilized application of molecular sonography involves a VEGF receptor antibody can be used as a ligand on a microbubble to detect tumor microvessels (**Figure 2**) [3]. This has shown to provide early detection of several cancers in murine models, notably pancreatic, prostate, and squamous cell carcinoma.

Labeled microbubbles may have an important role in monitoring tumor response to anti-angiogenic medications. In a preclinical proof of concept study using colon cancer models, 3D molecular sonography showed close correlation with treatment response to antiangiogenetic therapy [4].

Microbubble sonography can be used to assess the potential efficacy of specific anti-angiogenetic medications. In a pilot study of patients with refractory hepatocellular carcinomas, we found that a significant decrease in vascularity was seen in responsive vs. non-responsive tumors in the first 15 days after treatment was initiated (**Figure 3**) [5].

Similarly, molecular sonography has been studied as a means to evaluate acute ileitis in a swine model that targeted E- and P-selectin. The intensity of the sonographic signal correlated to the amount of immunofluorescence [6].

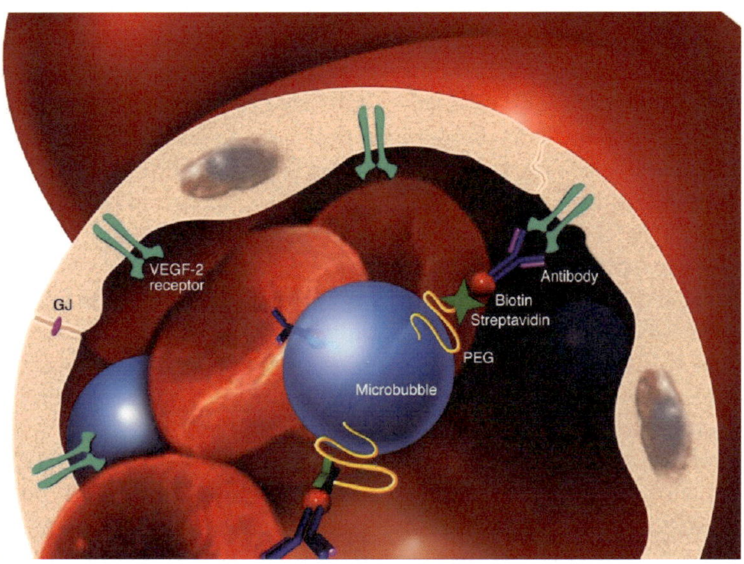

Figure 1.
Drawing showing the streptavidin/biotin spacer for attachment of anti-VEGF receptor to microbubble.

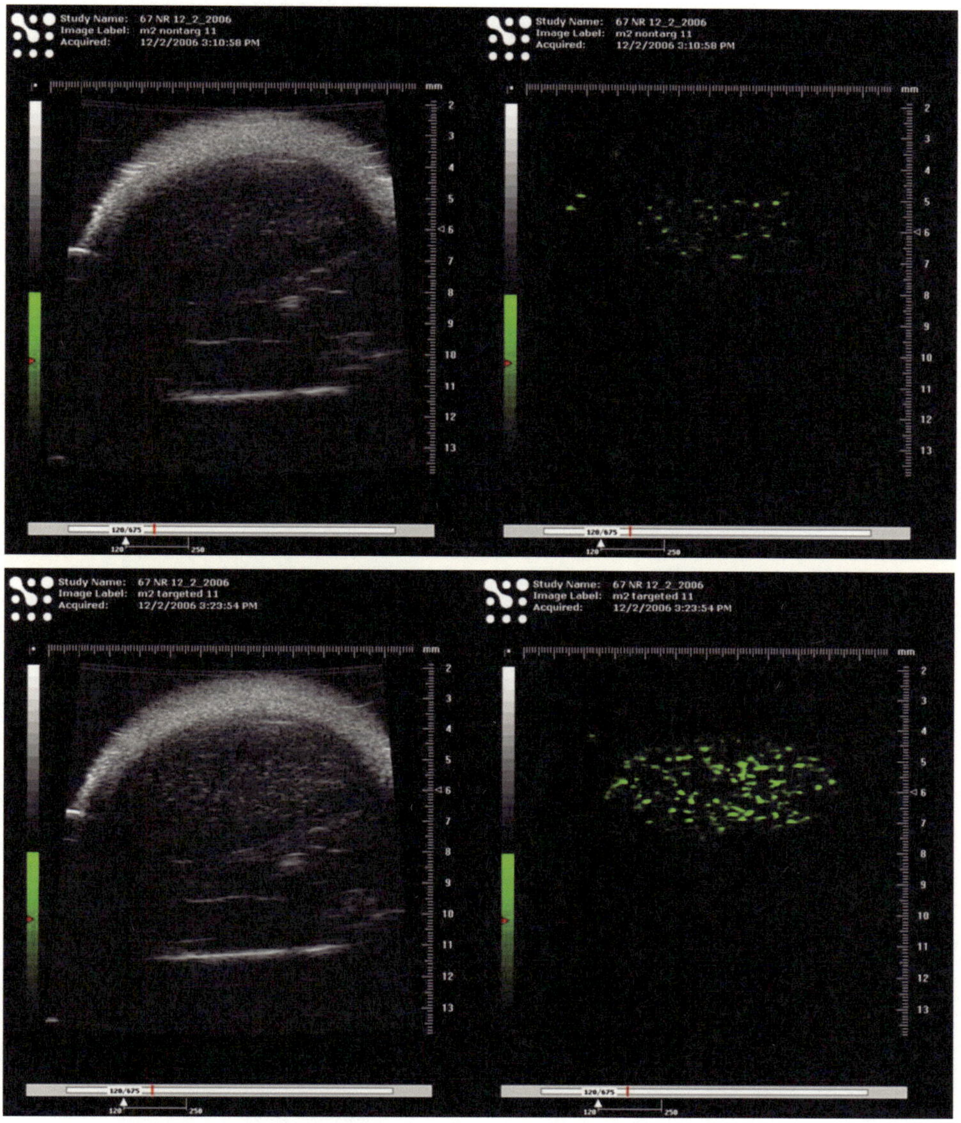

Figure 2.
Molecular sonograms of implanted murine tumor with low (top) and high (bottom) VEGF receptors as confirmed with immunofluorescence [2].

3. Potential clinical applications

The main potential clinical application of labeled microbubbles includes early detection of tumors, monitoring tumor response, assessment of inflammation and/or ischemia, early detection of transplant infection and potential for targeted drug delivery.

One of the challenges to use these microbubbles is their fabrication for clinical use. Specifically, the immunogenicity of the streptavidin used for attaching the ligand to the bubble requires that it be internalized within the microbubble. This is only available from a few manufacturers on an investigational basis. We reported our early experience developing a labeled microbubble [7].

Only a few studies using labeled microbubbles in humans have been reported [1]. The group headed by Willman showed that breast and ovarian malignant

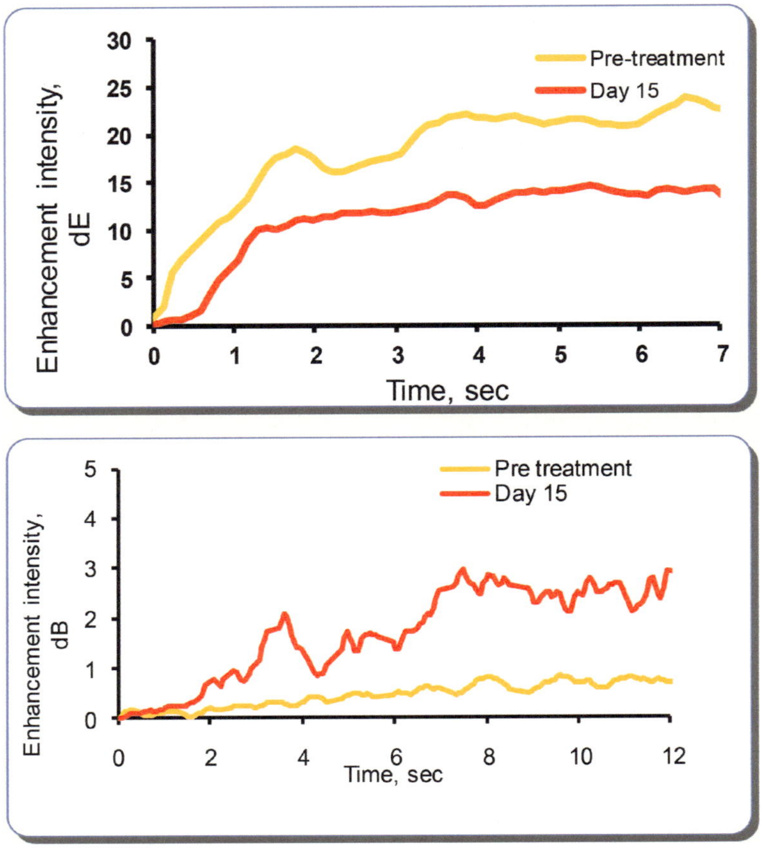

Figure 3.
Time intensity curve in responsive (top) vs. non-responsive (bottom) hepatocellular cancer treated with anti-angiogenic medications.

tumors had greater signal than benign ones. Specifically, in a study of 24 patients with ovarian cancers and 21 with breast lesions, 93% of malignant breast lesions and 77% of malignant ovarian cancers demonstrated increased signal [1].

Labeled microbubbles have also been used in detecting prostate cancer and sentinel lymph nodes [7, 8]. Molecular lymphosonography was used to detect metastatic involvement in a swine melanoma model. Metastatic involvement of the sentinel lymph node can distinguish local vs. metastatic disease in women with breast cancer. It has also been used in a variety of cancers such as melanoma, esophageal, head and neck, stomach and thyroid cancer. Molecular sonography using nanobubble targeted prostate specific membrane antigen has been investigated in an orthotopic murine model [8]. Increased extravasation and retention were observed in prostate cancer models as well as exhibiting different time/intensity curves (enhancement kinetics) in cancerous tissue.

Angiogenesis, the generation of new blood vessels, has also been extensively investigated with molecular sonography due to its role in the development and metastatic spread of numerous cancers. It is crucial in the growth of tumors and subsequent metastasis. VEGFR2 is one of the most studied markers of angiogenesis and is over expressed on tumor-associated endothelial cells [9]. In one study of a transgenic mouse model, microbubbles targeting VEGFR2 showed an increased contrast-enhanced ultrasound signal from hyperplasia to ductal carcinoma in situ and breast cancer compared to normal breast tissue [10]. In another study of laying hens, a microbubble targeting $\alpha v\beta 3$ integrin sensitively detected ovarian cancer at an early stage [11]. These are just two studies that support the clinical utility of angiogenesis targeted microbubbles in early tumor detection.

Applying the principles of molecular sonography to atherosclerosis can help identify at-risk plaques before acute events occur, potentially enabling prevention of evolution into irreversible damage. Normally, patients do not exhibit symptoms until an episode of severe stenosis or rupture occurs; thus, there is valuable utility in monitoring the growth of atherosclerotic plaques. JAM-A is an example of a marker that has been linked to early plaque formation and vulnerability [12]. In a study performed on mice that were fed an atherogenic diet, molecular ultrasound of JAM-A showed early stages of atherosclerosis and detected acute blood flow variations [13].

Acute cardiac ischemia is another pathology that would benefit from molecular ultrasound imaging. Current methods of detection such as EKG and cardiac MRIs suffer from various shortcomings such as accuracy, convenience, or safety. Sonography with labeled microbubbles could resolve a number of these shortcomings when used to identify post-ischemic myocardium. E- and P- selectin are two potential markers that were used in murine models to identify ischemic tissue shortly after undergoing an ischemic event [14, 15]. While cardiac molecular ultrasound imaging has shown promising results regarding safety and efficacy, it is technically difficult and highly user-dependent. Further testing needs to be performed to assess its feasibility when compared with current gold standards.

Microbubbles also can be applied in the assessment of inflammatory bowel disease (IBD). Two methods of assessing IBD are endoscopy and ultrasound. The former requires a procedure under anesthesia, while the latter is restricted by its relatively limited sensitivity. Molecular ultrasound holds clinical potential to serve as a complementary tool with high sensitivity in the imaging of IBD. One study utilized porcine tissue with terminal ileitis imaged with dual E- and P-selectin-targeted microbubbles. The study concluded that increased ultrasound signal correlated well with histologic grades of inflammation [16]. This study highlights selectin-targeted ultrasound's utility to serve as a high-sensitivity adjunctive tool for assessment of IBD in the clinical setting.

4. Conclusions

Molecular sonography has great potential as a means to detect early stages of a variety of cancers as well as a means to evaluate tumor response. It is anticipated that more widespread clinical use will occur in the next few years once these microbubbles become more readily available.

Acknowledgements

Dr. Andrej Lyshchik is thanked for his original work in this topic.

Conflict of interest

The authors declare no conflicts of interest.

Author details

Arthur Fleischer[1*] and Sai Chennupati[2]

1 Vanderbilt University Medical Center, Nashville, USA

2 Vanderbilt University School of Medicine, Nashville, USA

*Address all correspondence to: arthur.fleischer@vumc.org

References

[1] Willmann JK, Bonomo L, Testa AC, Rinaldi P, Rindi G, Valluru KS, et al. Ultrasound molecular imaging with br55 in patients with breast and ovarian lesions: First-in-human results. Journal of Clinical Oncology. 2017;35(19):2133-40. DOI: 10.1200/JCO.2016.70.8594

[2] Lyshchik A, Fleischer AC, Huamani J, Hallahan DE, Brissova M, Gore JC. Molecular imaging of vascular endothelial growth factor receptor 2 expression using targeted contrast-enhanced high-frequency ultrasonography. J Ultrasound Med. 2007;26(11):1575-1586. DOI:10.7863/jum.2007.26.11.1575

[3] Hwang M, Lyshchik A, Fleischer AC. Molecular sonography with targeted microbubbles: current investigations and potential applications. Ultrasound Q. 2010;26(2):75-82. DOI:10.1097/RUQ.0b013e3181df96de

[4] Zhou J, Wang H, Zhang H, Lutz AM, Tian L, Hristov D, et al. Vegfr2-targeted three-dimensional ultrasound imaging can predict responses to antiangiogenic therapy in preclinical models of colon cancer. Cancer Research. 2016;76(14):4081-9. DOI: 10.1158/0008-5472.CAN-15-3271

[5] Wang H, Hyvelin JM, Felt SA, et al. US Molecular Imaging of Acute Ileitis: Anti-Inflammatory Treatment Response Monitored with Targeted Microbubbles in a Preclinical Model. Radiology. 2018;289(1):90-100. DOI:10.1148/radiol.2018172600

[6] Pinkerton A, Fleischer AC. Early Detection of Type II Ovarian Cancer with Labelled Microbubble Transvaginal Sonography. J Gyn Women's Health, 2017:5:5-7. DOI:10.19080/JGWH.2017.05.555668

[7] Nam K, Stapp R, Liu JB, et al. Performance of Molecular Lymphosonography for Detection and Quantification of Metastatic Involvement in Sentinel Lymph Nodes. J Ultrasound Med. 2019;38(8):2103-2110. DOI:10.1002/jum.14906

[8] Wang, Y., De Leon, A., Perera, R. et al. Molecular imaging of orthotopic prostate cancer with nanobubble ultrasound contrast agents targeted to PSMA. Sci Rep 11, 4726 (2021). DOI:10.1038/s41598-021-84072-5

[9] Ferrara N. Vascular endothelial growth factor: basic science and clinical progress. Endocr Rev. 2004;25(4):581-611. doi:10.1210/er.2003-0027

[10] Bachawal SV, Jensen KC, Lutz AM, et al. Earlier detection of breast cancer with ultrasound molecular imaging in a transgenic mouse model. Cancer Res. 2013;73(6):1689-1698. DOI:10.1158/0008-5472.CAN-12-3391

[11] Barua A, Yellapa A, Bahr JM, et al. Enhancement of ovarian tumor detection with αvβ3 integrin-targeted ultrasound molecular imaging agent in laying hens: a preclinical model of spontaneous ovarian cancer. Int J Gynecol Cancer. 2014;24(1):19-28. DOI:10.1097/IGC.0000000000000040

[12] Babinska, A., Azari, B. M., Salifu, M. O., Liu, R., Jiang, X. C., Sobocka, M. B., Boo, D., Al Khoury, G., Deitch, J. S., Marmur, J. D., Ehrlich, Y. H., & Kornecki, E. (2007). The F11 receptor (F11R/JAM-A) in atherothrombosis: overexpression of F11R in atherosclerotic plaques. *Thrombosis and haemostasis*, *97*(2), 272-281.

[13] Curaj A, Wu Z, Rix A, et al. Molecular Ultrasound Imaging of Junctional Adhesion Molecule A Depicts Acute Alterations in Blood Flow and Early Endothelial Dysregulation. Arterioscler Thromb Vasc Biol. 2018;38(1):40-48. DOI:10.1161/ATVBAHA.117.309503

[14] Kaufmann BA, Lewis C, Xie A, Mirza-Mohd A, Lindner JR. Detection of recent myocardial ischaemia by molecular imaging of P-selectin with targeted contrast echocardiography. Eur Heart J. 2007;28(16):2011-2017. DOI:10.1093/eurheartj/ehm176

[15] Leng, X., Wang, J., Carson, A., Chen, X., Fu, H., Ottoboni, S., Wagner, W. R., & Villanueva, F. S. (2014). Ultrasound detection of myocardial ischemic memory using an E-selectin targeting peptide amenable to human application. *Molecular imaging*, *13*, 1-9.

[16] Wang H, Felt SA, Machtaler S, et al. Quantitative Assessment of Inflammation in a Porcine Acute Terminal Ileitis Model: US with a Molecularly Targeted Contrast Agent. Radiology. 2015;276(3):809-817. DOI:10.1148/radiol.2015142478